Read why thes
How To Ha

MW00438485

"If new parents want to have healthy children, they are facing challenges like never before. The rise of life-damaging diseases such as autism and allergies is alarming. The standard diet kids are eating is empty and toxic. Common medical procedures are often useless and sometimes dangerous. Money, rather than the wellbeing of children, is far too often the driving force behind policy and practices.

I urge parents and parents-to-be to buy and read Dr. Gemmer's vital message. It will show them new ways to look at these issues and provide the ideas needed to overcome today's obstacles and have healthy children."

Dr. Jack Wolfson, D.O., Fellow of the American College of Cardiology and Author of "The Paleo Cardiologist"

★   ★

"Parents from around the country are bringing their children to our practice in Dallas in ever increasing numbers, seeking help for their children with autism, ADD/ADHD, electromagnetic sensitivity, diabetes and allergies including severe food allergies and autoimmunity. Many are parents who don't want to see their children continually medicated.

Dr. Gemmer has done a phenomenal job of describing the problem with western medicine's evolution into treatment consisting of medicating symptoms instead of recognizing the CAUSES of these diseases. He educates parents on the dangers of the growing number of toxins in the environment and in everyday foods, and how these toxins cause disease.

This book is a valuable resource for any parent or parent-to-be who is intent on having healthy children in the face of so many obstacles, both political and environmental. Parents, PLEASE read this book. Your children are counting on you."

Stephanie McCarter MD - Environmental Health Center of Dallas. American Board of Internal Medicine Certified, Member of the American Academy of Environmental Medicine and Naturopathic Academy of Environmental Medicine

HOW TO HAVE
HEALTHY
CHILDREN

*In Spite of
Western Medicine,
Trashy Food and
Know-it-All Relatives*

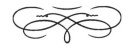

Dr. Erwin Gemmer

Contents

THIS BOOK SOLVES THESE PROBLEMS

FIRST AND FOREMOST, this book will help prevent your baby from being damaged by chemicals, toxins and procedures that *we are told* make babies healthier. Moms (and dads) who don't get this information are very likely to have their pregnancies complicated, see the delivery of their babies turned into disasters and then wonder where they went wrong as their babies develop lifelong problems.

After watching the staggering increases of childhood autism, diabetes, ADHD, allergies, asthma and even cancer, it is clear that something serious is wrong. Half the babies and children shouldn't be sick and diseased! You are rightly concerned regarding how to keep this from happening to your baby. But when you try to research "why" so many children get chronic diseases that start during childhood, you become buried in endless conflicting data.

In this book, you will finally find simple, obvious answers that make so much sense. You'll also learn that many of the most important things are what NOT to do and what not to allow.

One other big benefit of this book is that you will soon know how to handle the counter intentions and agendas of others. Once you fully understand what it takes to have a healthy baby, you will no longer have to tolerate pressure from doctors, nurses, school officials, friends, relatives or anyone else. You will *know* what you know, and if someone tries to treat you like you're stupid, you'll immediately be able to stop them dead in their tracks.

My goal is for you to have a wonderful pregnancy, low stress delivery, a healthy, happy baby and not take a beating in the process.

A NOTE REGARDING
THE CONTENT OF THIS BOOK

EVERYTHING CONTAINED IN THIS BOOK is for educational purposes, written here to help parents understand the many decisions they will need to make that will either enhance or damage the health of their child. Because Dr. Gemmer obviously doesn't know specific details regarding any one particular child, nothing in this book is offered to diagnose or treat any known or unknown disease, nor should this book be construed as a recommendation to stop or start any form of medical treatment. Before acting on any suggestions in this book, feel free to consult a doctor, the FDA, the AMA, the ACS, the CDC, the NIMH or the drug companies that spend hundreds of millions to make sure our children grow up dependent on as many drugs as possible. All content in this book is author's educated opinion only. You alone are responsible for decisions you make regarding your child.

PART I

How I Got Into
The "Healthy Baby" Battle

My Initiation Into
The World Of Denial

THE YEAR WAS 2008. I had for some time been accumulating information on vaccinations. To my surprise, most of the information from non-biased sources showed almost all the vaccinations to be dangerous, useless *or both*. I discovered the extremely poisonous nature of many of the vaccine ingredients. I learned that almost all the infectious diseases that we had been told were eradicated by vaccinations had in fact mostly gone away on their own *before the vaccinations were introduced.* I found that several of the most dangerous vaccines were repeatedly given to babies and toddlers at the worst possible ages.

The more I learned, the more I felt compelled to bring this information to the public. So my staff scheduled a program, "Vaccinations: Are They Safe or Effective?" at a local community center.

On the night of the event, dozens of concerned parents filled the room.

But to add a bit of spice to my life, we were blessed also by the presence of a local pediatrician. Now as I tell this story, keep in mind that without "well baby" visits (translation: healthy babies going to pediatricians for vaccinations), most pediatricians would be out of business literally overnight.

As the program progressed that evening, I proved one point after another through solid medical references and obvious logic. If mercury and aluminum were among the most dangerous nerve toxins on earth, how could it be safe to inject them multiple times into tiny babies? If formaldehyde causes cancer and if cancer is a major killer among children, why would we want to inject our infants with it? Why would baby be given three tetanus shots by age six months, when any immunity from them would fade away before baby could possibly step on a rusty nail? Also, if a baby was hundreds of times as likely to die from a tetanus shot as from tetanus, how could that possibly be a smart thing to give babies?

So here's what happened. Throughout the whole program, the pediatrician was again and again interrupting with comments and off-topic questions. Finally one of the men in attendance stood up and said, "We're all here to learn something and we would appreciate it if you would just shut up!" Everyone clapped. Awkward, right?

With my head on the pillow that night, I pondered what had happened at the presentation and why this pediatrician would clash head on against all the solid evidence, even to the point of embarrassing herself.

As I thought about this during the weeks that followed, I started to see the whole picture of what we were up against. This *one* local doctor was merely echoing misinformation that had meticulously been planted in her head throughout her schooling and career. What she *thought she knew* originated in the marketing departments of huge multi-national drug companies, those that view our kids as cash cows from which to extract money. These giant pharmaceutical companies are then assisted by government agencies, medical associations, certain professions and finally by the local practitioners. The big players in this process *are* actively seeking to make billions. If they happen to harm children in the process, that's collateral damage they're willing to live with, especially when this damage has a secondary effect of producing lifelong customers.

The medical associations and individual practitioners are simply and quietly going along with all that is occurring, choosing to turn a blind eye to the bad and pretending it isn't happening. But they are *all* part of it. And making money.

Once I saw all this for what it was, I knew that I had to speak up. It wasn't just *one* doctor under the influence of this misinformation campaign. It was almost *all* of them. Most, in turn, were then pounding parents with what they had been told to believe.

To counteract this assault, I realized that millions of parents needed concise information that wasn't tainted by financially motivated bias, not only about vaccinations but about everything related to pregnancy, delivery and early childhood. This certainly included information on what is wrong with the modern diet and how to safely feed children. I also became aware of how badly parents needed help defending themselves and their children from institutions, professions and corporations with profit-at-all-cost intentions. And all too often, from misled doctors and know-it-all relatives.

The real breakthrough came when I fully accepted one reality: all the wrong that doctors and parents are taught regarding babies and children can be traced directly to *money!*

For instance, do you think anyone over at General Mills or Kellogg's really believes breakfast cereals that are 50% sugar are "part of a nutritional breakfast?" Which part? The sugar? The ink used to color it? The fake flavors?

Is it possible that the people at the CDC and the American Pediatric Association can't see that kids were far healthier years ago with three or four vaccinations than they are now with well over 65?

Can obstetricians or hospitals possibly believe that 30% of all babies need to be delivered cesarean?

Money and profit appear to rule, no matter the collateral damage.

The Surprise Attack Parents Rarely See Coming

YOU KNOW THAT SOMETHING is wrong in a major way. You've seen the alarming statistics showing the number of kids sick with allergies, asthma, autism, diabetes, obesity and even cancer.

You suspect it is the degraded food. Or the dozens of questionable vaccinations. Or maybe even the way that babies are born.

But when you mention your suspicions, your doctor tells you that no one knows why the kids are so sick, that it is just a mystery. You tell a close friend or relative that you are thinking about not vaccinating your kids and they attack you like you're trying to start an epidemic.

You get lost in a world of indecision.

Then one day, you are forced to make an on-the-spot decision. "You need a cesarean delivery." Or "your two-month-old baby needs five vaccinations today." Or "the only way to stop these earaches is through antibiotics and putting tubes into your child's ears." Or "your son doesn't stand a chance in school without Ritalin."

Suddenly, there you are, with the authority figures pressing you to do something you feel in your heart isn't right. Should you disagree? Make a scene? Who are you to challenge the "experts" anyway?

If you haven't run up against this type of situation, you will. And when you do, your baby's only safety net is for you to really be prepared for it.

Here's what happens: a couple takes their baby to the clinic. They think that the staff will check their little baby and tell them everything is going great. The clinic, however, has a totally different agenda. They fully intend to give this two-month-old baby seven vaccinations.

Now maybe these parents have heard that these vaccines contain mercury, aluminum, formaldehyde, acetone, latex, antibiotics, animal DNA and more, and don't see how putting these poisons into their eight-pound baby could possibly be safe. Or perhaps their friends were talked into giving their baby these same shots, and the little one then screamed day and night for the next week.

So these parents have the idea that they don't want these shots, that they will say, "NO!" That's their intention.

But . . . right then is when it happens. Everyone in this clinic has been drilled on how to overpower each and every objection that these parents might think of and a bunch of others besides. So as this "Well Baby" visit progresses, these parents are shamed and bullied into submission. They finally cave in and sign the release forms.

Do you think this is a rare occurrence? Not even close! This happens a hundred thousand times every week! The parents showing up at the clinic with their baby is like little Bambi strolling through a forest during hunting season.

So, parents and parents-to-be, this book is for you. You will soon be armed with the information you need to make all the key decisions, in advance, so you won't be caught unprepared and ambushed into doing something you're pretty sure isn't in your baby's best interest.

I should mention here that I could fill a dozen pages with a serious bibliography and support all statements from multiple sources. However,

I choose not to because this book was written for those with common sense, those who think.

For those who would insist on seeing a double-blind study before they'd believe water is wet or that gravity makes things fall, this book may not be a fit. However, if you are willing to use your logic and reason as you read, you'll soon discover that this book describes *exactly* what is occurring and what you may want to consider instead if you want to keep your children away from a very toxic, deceptive, for-profit, disease-causing system.

The Facts Today:
Children Aren't Healthy

HERE'S THE SITUATION: in America, we have entire drug and food related industries making billions of dollars pushing products and procedures that they know cause diseases. And worse yet, some of these same industries later go on to make billions more treating the diseases they caused.

I don't think there are any cases on record where either the pharmaceutical industry or the "food" companies intentionally set out to harm children. But what they have done many hundreds of times is to bring drugs and "foodish" products to market. With each new drug or product, they hope for a blockbuster, one that will first bring in tens of millions and hopefully eventually billions of dollars. Free enterprise at work!

But then comes the dilemma. When it is found that this drug or that product is causing lifelong diseases in children, what should these giant corporations do then? Pull the product off the market and cause the company profits to plummet while angering the stockholders and getting the CEO fired? Or . . . should they look the other way and keep on selling it?

Unfortunately, the "keep on selling it" option is usually chosen. Then, as dangers of this drug or product receive more and more attention, they stoop even lower and begin cover-up operations. One good lie deserves another. So they double down and do whatever it takes to keep the profits flowing.

Another unfortunate fact today is that far too often, pregnancy and childbirth are looked upon as if they were "diseases" that need medical intervention. This same meddling continues through baby's first years. At every step, it is assumed that medical interventions are needed, with each of them in turn causing a cascade of ill effects that bring about the need for other harmful interventions. The more that this is done, the worse it gets!

Think about it: unless parents put a stop to it, by the time babies are two years old, they will have had 20 or 30 vaccinations laced with extracts from cow, pig, monkey and chicken as well as latex, antibiotics, mercury, aluminum, acetone, formaldehyde and other brain-damaging, cancer-causing poisons. And another 30 or 40 poison-ladened vaccinations are waiting right around the corner, all of which *will* be injected by age twelve *if parents allow it!*

These vaccinations for kids are aggressively pushed upon their un-suspecting parents. The CDC alone gets over two billion dollars per year from the taxpayers to promote vaccination. Do you think that much money might encourage someone somewhere do unscrupulous things?

With the same wild abandon, unnecessary surgeries are done on young children to the point where they are commonplace, even routine. Other than making money, there's no good reason for doing them.

On and on it goes.

What is the overall result of all this money grabbing nonsense?

In a word, the answer is: DISEASE.

Take autism for example. You start with a perfectly healthy baby. He or she is developing normally, interacting with parents and siblings, is outgoing, smiling and interested.

Then, almost overnight, this child stops communicating and regresses into a mental and emotional prison. While some people with autism function at a high level, about 25% have an IQ of 70 or below. Somewhere around 40% of autistics will never function independently. Many make loud, incoherent noises, and may thrash about violently, even injuring those attempting to care for them.

Autism victims and their families are never the same.

Autism used to be rare. In fact, it was unknown until 1943 when a well know physician observed a neurological condition, never seen before, in 11 kids.

Since then, autism occurrences have skyrocketed, literally increasing from one in a million kids to currently about 1 in 50 children between the age of 3 and 17 in the U.S alone.

There are already approximately 500,000 people with autism that function at a very low level. The cost to care for each of them has been calculated to be between $1,000,000 and $2,500,000 over a lifetime. The total cost? If you do the math, you'll find that the cost of just those who *already* have been given autism is a TRILLION dollars! And many more are on the way.

There are at least 200 times as many cases of autism today as there were 45 years ago. Two hundred times! What is even more shocking is that the big shots who are watching these alarming numbers act like they don't know what is causing autism.

And cancer. *Many* children get cancer. In fact, in the United States, cancer is the second leading cause of death in all kids ages 5 through 15, surpassed only by deaths due to accidents. Again, most of the causes are rather obvious; therefore, most cases could almost certainly be prevented. But is anyone talking about prevention?

And obesity. Roughly a third of today's children are overweight (many are *very* overweight), and far too many of them have diabetes or are well on their way to having it. To offer some idea how big this situation is, almost half of all Americans have diabetes or are pre-diabetic. The trends are far more frightening than what we are seeing today based on the direction our children are headed.

And asthma and allergies. Staggering numbers of children have asthma or allergies. Common foods that have kept humans alive for centuries now throw these kids into life-threatening reactions. Doesn't that seem odd to you?

Is all this accidental? Does it "just happen" and no one can explain why? Or . . . are the causes of these diseases now known *but* both the causes *and* the diseases are simply too profitable to abandon?

You will soon know and have certainty.

Who Am I And
How Did I Get Here?

WHILE ATTENDING A SEMINAR recently, a young woman asked what I did. When I told her I trained new moms and soon-to-be moms (and dads) how to get baby started right, she looked a little puzzled.

She said I didn't look like a midwife, definitely didn't look like a mom. Obstetrician perhaps? Nope.

So why me writing this book?

I am a natural healthcare provider and educator. For over 40 years, I've taught moms and dads how to have healthy babies and children in spite of being misled by misguided doctors, in spite of all the toxic foods, and even in spite of the various dangerous vaccinations. I've helped parents prevent diseases and sicknesses in their children. Originally trained as a chiropractor, my studies have expanded on that many times since. I'm also the father of 10 extremely healthy children.

Throughout four decades, my studies focused on how to be healthy naturally. However, as the years went by, it became more and more evident that we needed to focus far more of our attention on the time around pregnancy, delivery and childhood. Why? Because millions of children are damaged *early* and then suffer from that damage *the rest of their lives.*

But what *really* motivated me to write this book is that, in most all cases, this damage could have been prevented by parents simply knowing a few basics and making some key decisions.

I've attended many dozens of seminars and put on hundreds more, teaching thousands what I've learned over the years. When attendees learn that I have so many children, the next question is usually, "Are you Catholic? Or Mormon?" Sorry to disappoint anyone, but I'm neither.

Were the kids all planned? Nope. None of them!

But my experiences and all the children certainly have given me plenty of reasons to study what it takes to get babies started right. And what can go wrong.

As I've helped parents learn about all the ways their babies can potentially be damaged, they commonly wonder at first, "What IS ok? What CAN my children safely eat? Who CAN we really believe (or trust)?"

The answer really comes down to one basic truth: the more that someone believes we should muddle things up by working against nature (a doctor, perhaps), the less you should trust him/her. And conversely, the more someone truly understands that the innate mechanisms built into all of us to promote health and survival rarely make mistakes, the wiser you'd be to follow *their* lead.

For instance, let's say we have two basic options regarding what goes into your toddler:

Option 1 is clean air, pure water and simple, naturally grown food.

Option 2 is air and water loaded with pollutants, along with processed "food" that has been sprayed with poisons in the field and then poisoned again and again later with preservatives, artificial sweeteners and colors, synthetic vitamins and all the rest.

OK, which is better for a young child? Option 1? Or Option 2?

An easy choice, right? And it is easy because, no matter what the question, the best answer is always the same: WORK WITH NATURE.

Picture this scene: a mom was told that she needed some special procedure during her delivery. Or that baby needed drugs, shots or a surgery. Maybe she was pushed to do this. Maybe she was uninformed and just went along. Or perhaps it didn't seem like a very big deal at the time.

Instead of this procedure helping, things went badly as is very often the case, and baby was damaged. Now the parents are wondering how to undo the injuries and damage. They wish they had their healthy, happy baby back.

But it's not likely to fully occur. The damage is done. It's like breaking a lamp or a vase and trying to glue it back right. It's just never the same.

I don't want this for you or your baby. And, I don't want this situation to continue to play out thousands and thousands of times every day like it does now.

PART II

HOW DID WE EVER GET INTO SUCH A MESS?

Back Then Versus Right Now

WHEN I WAS IN GRADE SCHOOL, there wasn't a single kid in our entire school allergic to anything. But now? Allergies run rampant through our young population.

Asthma was rare. Now there are a couple kids in every class who can't leave home without their steroid inhalers. They get asthma when they are young and keep it for a lifetime.

Back then, you had to smoke three packs of cigarettes a day for forty years to get cancer, and there really was only about one type of cancer, lung cancer. In contrast, cancer is now a leading cause of death in kids.

Fifty years ago, a very few kids were overweight. In fact, reflecting on the school I attended, I can think of only five who were overweight out of close to 300 students (and they were so rare, I can still *name* them now, more than 50 years later). But now in the same age group? In most places, at least one-fourth of the kids are overweight, and in some schools, it's closer to one-third.

As I mentioned a couple of chapters back, only a handful of children used to have autism. Numbers just in from New Jersey (the worst state in America) say that one out of 23 boys now has autism there. And this trend is absolutely not slowing. The numbers are worse every year.

How about this for major, underreported situation: girls are starting their female cycle in the second and third grades! By the time they are

11, most girls are as developed as their moms were when they graduated from high school. Nobody's talking about it. And worse, no one is asking the obvious question: "WHY?"

We are looking at staggering increases and lifelong problems.

As parents who are concerned and seek answers, we are insulted by the ridiculous explanations the authorities and "experts" offer for these huge increases in childhood disease, whether it's cancer, asthma, autism, autoimmunity or any one of the others.

One of the most laughable "reasons" we are given is that it is genetic, as if bad genes *on their own* suddenly kicked into gear in the last generation and started causing all of this after NOT causing any of it for the thousands of years before.

Sure, that makes a lot of sense. Why didn't we think of that?

So, what on earth is really going on?

Well, the most important thing a person needs to absolutely know is that ALL OF THIS IS CAUSED! There are always reasons why! Things don't just happen.

But instead of looking for the cause, we are supposed to believe in what I call the "boogie man" theory of disease, which goes like this: a kid is just going through life, minding his own business, perfectly healthy and then WHAM! Cancer. Or autism. Or diabetes.

Who can explain it? It's just bad luck, right?

That is utter nonsense! Things are CAUSED. As I already mentioned, most of this is being caused by things which are occurring very early in life, during childbirth or the early years.

Yes, child after child, the health crisis starts early in life.

To understand why I'd say that, we must look at how foods and medicine got to where they are now from where they were back then.

ṣ Sixth Chapter ṣ

How Food Became Depleted and Poisoned

WHEN I WAS A CHILD in the 1950's, our family lived on a small farm, as did most families in North America and around the world. We had three cows, a couple dozen chickens, a huge garden, numerous types of berries and orchard trees that produced nuts and fruits. The soil was alive with bugs and worms, and was allowed to "rest" and replenish several months of the year. It was further fed through application of compost and animal manure.

Looking back now, I realize I didn't appreciate the value of all this. Imagine, every mineral on earth readily available for the crops and the animals that foraged in the fields. The food that grew there was second to none. The fresh eggs, milk, butter, beef and chicken were rich sources of nutrition. The same was true of all the plant crops.

But about this same time, a change began to occur. Chemical farming was born.

Farmers were encouraged to dose their fields with chemical fertilizers which consisted of only three elements, nitrogen, potassium and phosphorus. While these three elements would grow big, lush-appearing crops, no one noticed that the plants were gradually starved of the other

60 or 70 things that they had previously gotten from the soil. This situation was worsened as the farms began to produce two or three crops per year in warmer climates.

Because all of this made the plants sick, they became susceptible to pests. Conveniently, the same industries that produced the chemical fertilizer then "came to the rescue" with pesticides and fungicides. Soon all the bugs and worms in the soil were killed. The number of bees, birds and butterflies available to pollinate the crops was reduced dramatically.

As this continued year after year, the soil became more and more depleted. The field crops got sicker and therefore more susceptible to pests. Ever increasing tons of toxic chemicals were sprayed in an effort to kill everything that could attack the weakened plants.

We then ate the yield of these crops. We also ate the animal products from cattle, pigs and chickens that ate these crops.

During these same transition years, most of the families gradually moved off their farms, usually for homes in the suburbs and jobs in the cities. Few of them noticed the change that was taking place in the food. As they bought more and more of their food in the stores and kept on eating it as if nothing had changed, they didn't realized they were gradually being starved of key nutrients and consuming larger and larger amounts of toxins.

As a result, these years saw a huge increase in diseases caused by nutritional deficiencies and subtle poisoning.

But something far worse was soon to come.

In 1994, the first genetically engineered (GE) and genetically modified organism (GMO) products arrived in the stores. The concept of GMO's is to add genes from one species of plant or animal into the genes of a crop plant. For instance, if a certain plant or animal could tolerate cold weather, wouldn't adding its genes to a plant that was prone to frost damage be a good thing? It seemed OK at first.

However, we now know there are at least three reasons GE and GMO foods set us up for a disaster of epic proportions.

First, as bacterial genes are injected into the genetic code of corn, it makes it so the corn doesn't just *contain* a pesticide. It *becomes* a pesticide!

That's right, genes are spliced into corn so that the corn grows pesticides right into the kernels, poisons that will kill any pest that attempts to eat it. The problems is, it is still there poisoning anything that eats it *after it is harvested*, people for example.

To give you an idea of how poisonous this corn is and how this might apply to you as an expectant mother or a new parent, more than half the offspring of pregnant rats that eat this corn die. Additionally, when this corn is eaten by us (or we eat anything that has eaten this corn such as pork or beef), it causes death and/or mutations of the friendly bacteria that live in our intestines. Trillions of them. Ruined. Inflammation, sickness, poor immunity, horrible digestive problems, allergies. These are just a few of the outcomes.

Remember, we're not just talking about directly eating corn. All these same problems are caused by consuming corn sweeteners, high fructose corn syrup, snack chips, candy, soda and a thousand other things people today commonly eat and drink.

Second, Roundup-tolerant wheat and soy are engineered so they can handle quantities of Roundup weed poison and its active ingredient, Glyphosate, multiple times per crop. Roundup goes right into the wheat and soy plants. The wheat and soy manage to live and for now, the weeds die. But crop after crop, year after year, more Roundup is sprayed on the fields. Ever increasing amounts get into the grain and beans, and build up in the soil, making the situation progressively worse. There is little doubt Roundup causes cancer and changes human hormone levels, unfortunate facts considering 5 billion pounds have already been dumped onto American farmland, and four times that much worldwide.

Once this poison is in the soil, it gets into everything else planted in that soil for decades (or maybe *centuries*).

Third is what happens with GMO sugar beets and the Roundup used as each sugar beet crop is grown. White sugar from *any* source and corn syrup from *all manner of* corn have each been a huge problem for at least 50 years. But now both are ALSO laced with toxic levels of Glyphosate. As it builds up in the soil, the toxic effects are worse with every passing year. Think of the implications, with Americans on average drinking 56 gallons of soda per year and with children drinking more than this average. Diabetes. Obesity. Cancer. Heart disease. Poor immunity. Digestive distress. Poor attention in school.

These diseases are all caused.

To further complicate the whole issue, after a few years, not even Bayer's (Monsanto's) mutated seeds will grow in the fields. The soil becomes so poisoned that it's difficult to get anything to grow there. Also, eventually weeds "find a way", and we then see weeds thriving in the toxic dirt while food crops planted there don't stand a chance. (Note: Bayer is not the only company selling mutilated seeds or toxic farm chemicals. It is just the biggest.)

Informed doctors are now finding that few kids have food allergies that aren't caused by either poisons in the foods or ingredients in vaccinations.

Here's another scary possibility: During the entire existence of humans on earth, plants have given us all ten of the essential amino acids needed to build proteins and strong bodies. But it appears the genetic changes in some GMO plants cause them to *make only half of these essential building blocks*. Kids (and their parents) depending on these for food may be starved of the basic materials needed to make and maintain cells of our bodies. While you ponder the implications of this, keep in mind that humans replace about 70 billion cells per day, and these cells are made from food. Without the building materials needed to replace every one of these cells, it is going to be a quick walk off a short plank.

How prevalent is Roundup in foods that aren't specifically labeled "non GMO?" Check this out: An independent lab tested over 70 oat-based baby and child products such as Cheerios, baby formula, canned baby food, granola, instant baby hot oatmeal, etc. All but two contained Roundup!

Corn, soybeans, sugar beets and wheat aren't the only genetically modified foods in the stores. Zucchini and summer squash, papaya, tomatoes, farmed salmon, canola oil, pineapple, potatoes, strawberries and alfalfa (fed to beef and dairy cows) are among the list of rogue toxic products. Additionally, the rBST hormones added to milk (see chapter 31), the synthetic sweetener aspartame and several artificial flavorings are all from genetically modified sources.

As a final fact for you to consider, pigs, chickens, salmon and cows that eat GMO corn, wheat or soy *concentrate these poisons* between 50 and 100 fold in their meat. Are they safe for you or your children to eat? No! Under no circumstance are they safe to eat.

Another Huge Change:
Birth With Violence

A SECOND HUGE SHIFT took place somewhere about 80 years ago. At that time, there was a massive transition in how babies were delivered, especially in developed, modern countries.

At that time, childbirth became a surgical procedure!

Now I want to stop you right here for a moment and let that soak in. Ponder just how weird of a change this really was. After thousands of years and hundreds of millions of babies, all the sudden it now took a surgical team to get the job done??

And wow, what a mess this change made of things.

An expectant mom is rushed to the hospital as if she'd just been shot in the chest. When she arrives, she is placed flat on her back on a hard, surgical table. She is strapped down, knocked out, given a paralyzing shot in the spine with her legs put up into stirrups and clamped in place.

When it's convenient for the doctor, he comes in, picks up a big set of steel tools like those you'd use to take a tire off a truck wheel. With these giant salad tongs, he grabs the baby's delicate little head and pulls and twists and yanks on the baby. The baby's neck is stretched to twice its normal length with the force you'd use if you were trying to uproot a small tree.

So many babies harmed . . .

You'd think once baby is fully winched out, dazed, drugged, damaged and confused, things couldn't get much worse. However, this is just the first of several colossal blunders.

Next, our tiny newborn baby's umbilical cord is cut far too soon, which instantly shuts off most of its oxygen.

Then, as baby starts turning blue from the disaster the obstetrician has caused, the doctor in a panic grabs the baby by an ankle or two, dangles the poor little thing upside down and spanks its wet rear to make it cry out in pain, thereby essentially forcing it to take its first breath.

To get an idea of what this was like for all of us babies back then, picture right now you are stripped naked, sprayed down with cold water and strapped upside down on the most extreme roller coaster, and then having your rear whipped as you flew through the air upside down for the next 40 seconds. Yeah, like that.

Mom is then "out" for several hours, maybe even a day or two. Baby is whisked away down the hall and kept warm like French fries waiting to be served.

Do you suppose baby feels alone and scared, wondering where he or she is? I don't really know. But I do know that as soon as a puppy or a colt or even a duck is born, it wants to bond with a parent. But no parents were around, not even dad because he "might get germs on the baby", you know.

Our poor baby is still drugged from the toxins which have passed through from mom. When the drugs finally wear off a bit, baby is hungry. But what to eat? Mom can't nurse because she still needs to be drugged due to all the pain caused by being cut, torn and sewn by the surgeon.

As a result, baby is fed corn syrup and water. Back then, in fact, parents were even told by their doctors this sugar water was better than breast milk.

Ok, great . . . it's been two or three days. Baby and mom finally go home. But is all the nonsense over once they exit (escape?) the hospital?

Nope. Later down the line, when kids got to be about four or five years old, into the hospital they'd go again, this time for the ritual of having their tonsils and adenoids cut out of their throats. Complete insanity? Certainly! But this was standard back then, and done on 1,200,000 kids the year I turned five.

Through these same years, doctors also started prescribing antibiotics to every kid who was at all sick, whether there was a hint of a bacterial infection or not. This blunder made the kids susceptible to *everything*. The thinking then (apparently) was that bacteria were bad and needed to be killed. Parents were encouraged to boil everything that could get near their babies and rinse dishes and silverware with a generous splash of chlorine bleach after they were washed. This germaphobic attitude prevailed then, and continues today as ordinary germs are coaxed into becoming super germs. Remember, with all the weaker bacteria killed and out of the picture, only the truly bad ones remain to multiply and fill the void.

Over time, tonsillectomy surgeries went out of style a bit. In fact, over the span of many years, it got to a point where only about half as many kids "needed" to have their "sick" tonsils cut out.

But then, surgeons instead busied themselves cutting the perfectly healthy appendix out of tens of thousands of kids each year. And then putting tubes in the ears. And then . . .

In the midst of all this, fetal monitors arrived on the birth scene, and a whole new chapter of ridiculous and unnecessary opened.

Mom was still placed on her back in the delivery room which, by the way, *always* cuts off much of the oxygen supply to the baby. But with the new fetal monitors, the surgical team saw what they had been causing all along, that laying mom on her back during delivery caused baby to be oxygen-deprived and in distress.

Did they simply sit mom up? Nope, that would be too easy. Instead, the delivery room crews went into panic mode. Code blue, code blue! We need to get this baby out fast!

Doctors started doing cesarean sections with a vengeance. Within a few years, many hospitals and doctors were doing cesarean deliveries 30 or 40% of the time. In fact, some doctors did ONLY cesareans!

On and on and on went all this nonsense and unnecessary intervention.

Continuity Of Craziness

So HERE WE ARE TODAY and here's my big question for you: do you think all the insanity is now gone? Do you think it just up and stopped? No, I wouldn't count on it.

The truth is, *much of what we have now is even more dangerous than what went on before.*

What does all this mean for you? First, all of the unnecessary intervention is harmful or dangerous, or at a minimum, useless. And because of it, the health, the wellbeing, the future of your baby or young child is at risk.

But here's the really great news for you: by you simply knowing a few basic things with absolute certainty, you can significantly increase the likelihood of the opposite, a healthy, happy baby *and* reduced chances of lifelong disease.

Now I want to clear something up right here. Do we *know* that the standard western medical birth process will end in baby being diagnosed with some sort of permanent damage? Do we *know* that unnecessary vaccinations will result in a diagnosed brain or immunity disease? Will child for certain react visibly to toxic GMO foods? Is baby *for sure* going to get autism or diabetes or cancer or asthma or allergies (or any of a dozen other serious conditions) from all this nonsense?

No, absolutely not. We do not know that.

However, we also don't know that a person who smokes for years will be diagnosed with lung or heart disease. Nope. Don't know that either. Truth is, while all smokers are obviously harmed, some of them manage to dodge the bullet long enough that they are never diagnosed with a smoking-related condition or disease.

Despite that, if it seems smart for a teen or adult to not smoke and thereby reduce the risk of disease and death, doesn't it similarly make sense to improve your baby's opportunities for health by keeping your little one away from things that are logically dangerous and damaging?

We all do this today in *some* areas of baby's life. For instance, we carefully place babies in backward-facing car seats to reduce injuries in case there's a wreck. Later, as babies grow a little older, we make sure they wear bicycle helmets to prevent brain damage in case of a hard fall.

But think of how many of these same babies were *already* seriously injured through unnecessary trauma in the delivery room as they were being born. Or how many already had their brains damaged 30 or more times from the mercury, aluminum, acetone and formaldehyde in vaccinations, all long before learning to ride a bike. Or poisoned by toxins in their food.

The Real Scoundrels

So AGAIN, WHY DO so many kids have asthma and diabetes and cancer? Why is it that kids can no longer eat wheat and peanuts and eggs and cheese and all the other foods that have kept humans alive for thousands of years? Why is it that 10% of American kids now supposedly have ADHD?

I'm going to repeat what I said before: asthma, diabetes, birth defects, ADHD, allergies, Crohn's disease, obesity, autoimmune disease, preteen cancer, autism . . . *ALL* of these things are CAUSED.

But here's the really disappointing (criminal) part: even when it is known what is causing each of these diseases, those who are causing them don't stop. Those who could expose them and blow the whistle *DON'T.* Those in charge of policing the whole situation look the other way. If they take any action at all, it is usually to misdirect or outright lie, sacrificing the health of millions of kids so profits keep rolling in.

Despite all the failures of the organizations that we associate with various diseases to teach true *prevention* (American Cancer Society, for instance), the one thing they *never* forget is to ask for tens of millions so they can search for a "cure."

Consider this: you would think that once it became known that one certain childhood vaccination increased the incidence of diabetes by 60%, there would have been a loud outcry from the Diabetes Association. But no, they haven't pressured the vaccine makers to modify or discontinue that shot. In fact, there's no evidence they are even vaguely interested. But they do want you to send money.

Or did you know that infants who are given antibiotics for earaches are three times as likely to have ear infections in the future? Despite this, the standard practice of giving antibiotics to kids for earaches remains unchanged.

Wouldn't you think someone at the Cerebral Palsy Foundation might want to know why countries where the birth process is less traumatic have a proportionally lower incidence of cerebral palsy?

Or does it seem important to you that 70% of all Crib Death (SIDS) cases in the United States occur within the three weeks following one certain vaccination, or that there is an eight-fold increase in infant deaths during the three days following this same vaccination? If this does seem important to you, you're in the minority. The CDC shows no interest whatsoever, and neither do the pharmaceutical companies or your local pediatricians.

Why is it that since 1986, the vaccination industry is the only industry in the world that is protected by the government from lawsuits arising from the hundreds of thousands of injuries and thousands of deaths caused by their toxic products?

Are the autism associations interested in why most other modern countries around the world have only a fraction of the autism cases found in the US? Or why the Amish here in America have *NONE?*

What government agency is asking why babies taken in for "Well Baby" pediatric visits are significantly sicker than those who aren't?

Also, ponder this: why isn't the American Cancer Society with its billion-dollar-a-year budget loudly telling us all the CAUSES of childhood cancer which, as I stated before, is the second leading cause of childhood death? I don't have a billion-dollar budget, yet I can list six causes of childhood cancers in the next half minute.

My Confession:
I Was Part Of The Problem

LOOK, I'VE BEEN WHERE you are. I went through all these same questions regarding medical procedures and toxic foods (and the diseases they cause) when my own children were young. We were seeking answers to these questions,

wondering what is right and which route we should take with each of our children. I put a lot of time into studying the research and pondering these questions.

All ten of my own children made it through. Their births were natural with no surgical teams. None of them got tubes put in their ears. No unnecessary vaccinations. No antibiotics. No tonsillectomies.

Just healthy, happy kids.

I've also had thousands of young parents and their kids as patients. As I got to know their stories and their health problems, one thing kept bothering me. I learned how parents were pressured to do things that weren't one bit necessary. I listened to them as they related how they were scared into having a cesarean delivery, "sold" on how their kids needed tubes in their ears, prescribed unnecessary antibiotic treatment when there was no infection and shamed into giving their infants vaccinations for conditions their baby couldn't possibly get.

For a long time when I heard this stuff, my immediate reaction was to say, "They wanted to do WHAT?? Why would they do that? Did you let them?"

I realized, though, that I was part of the problem because, even though I knew, *I hadn't told them what I knew.*

I also realized something else: the best time for parents to learn all about how to have a healthy baby was months (or even *years*) before they needed the information. Since then, I've guided many, many parents safely through this minefield of pregnancy, delivery and baby's early years.

Unfortunately, we live in a system dominated by western medicine, manufactured food, industrial chemical agricultural practices and aggressive marketing. As a result, all of our kids are truly at risk.

I want to help you avoid the wrong turns that can severely damage your child's health and immunity. And reduce the chances of childhood cancer. And allergies, asthma, Crohn's disease, autism, ADHD and crib death.

I am certain that well over 90% of ALL these diseases are preventable if we will *simply stop doing the things that are causing them.*

As I stated earlier, the organizations that should be doing the whistle-blowing aren't. But worse, some individuals in these groups have conflicts of interest of epic proportion, having been "purchased" by millions of dollars of "persuasion" money. Frankly, they lie, deceive, distort and misdirect. The rare individuals who dare to tell the truth watch helplessly as their careers and reputations are crushed.

So instead of these groups, organizations and agencies teaching all of us what is causing autism or cancer or asthma, and through this teaching prevention, they are telling us to "send money!" so they can look for a cure. Unfortunately, even if a cure did exist, it costs hundreds of times more to *attempt* to cure something than it would cost to simply prevent it. On top of this, as we all know, Western medical treatments almost always cause additional disease processes that in turn will need to be treated, which will in turn cause still more problems.

And around and around it goes.

Not even hundreds of millions of dollars will stop these diseases because, for them to be stopped, we would need people at the top who truly want health more than they want immense profits. Also remember, if somehow these diseases ever went away, the associations and professions making money off them would be out of business. That's just the way it is.

So, if you as a parent want to have the healthiest child possible, YOU will need to learn some things *and* be prepared to take a stand.

YOU Are What Makes
All The Difference

I KNOW THAT MILLIONS of new and expectant parents sense something is wrong. They have questions. They know this CAN'T be how things are supposed to be. They've been left in the dark. They struggle to find answers and then all too often get caught in the crosshairs after they've waited too long to find them.

If you are thinking about having a baby, I want you to be armed *in advance* with the right information to protect the health of your child and to take control of their future health. Also, I'd like you and millions of others to be prepared to say "NO!" when necessary, whether it is at the grocery or the pediatrician's office.

As a parent, you obviously want what's best for your child, so together let's drill down deep. You will soon discover there are relatively small numbers of choices which make all the difference, choices that determine whether a child will be healthy and disease-free or will struggle for a lifetime with problems that are difficult if not impossible to reverse.

The best time to get a map is before you go into the forest. Same with having a healthy child: it's so much better to KNOW before you GO!

PART III

———

WHAT IS A
NORMAL BIRTH?

Saved By The Sixties

WE MIGHT HAVE NEVER again known what a normal birth was were it not for one important and fortunate event: in the 1960's (and into the 1970's), a new group of thinkers appeared. They questioned about everything. Government. War. Religion. Rules. Gas guzzling cars. Chemical agriculture. Garbage. Worldly possessions and . . . *Medical authority.*

Keep in mind that before this time of questioning, the medical field and the obstetrical specialty were male dominated. Worse, their domination had a very "king of the castle" feel to it. Women would get dressed up to go to the doctor's office where they would often wait two or more hours for their appointment. Finally, they would be taken to a room and told by a nurse to strip. After sitting on a cold exam table for another half hour, the doctor would come in, reeking of smoke. Women simply weren't treated very well by doctors.

However, when this questioning and rebellion arrived in the 1960's, this acceptance of the doctor as the ultimate authority went out the window to a large degree. In its place came a gradual return to common sense. For the first time in decades, natural childbirth was an option.

The Normal Childbirth Sequence

As WE MOVE FORWARD here together, please keep in mind that there are many variables in childbirth, and no two births are the same. But it would be worth our time to now consider what a most-ideal delivery would be like.

First, mom would either stay in her usual environment (home) or go to a place that was happy, relaxed and quiet. She wouldn't be rushed or scared. She would go into the delivery with the confidence of knowing that many millions have done this before, it will be painful for a while, it will most likely be quite exhausting, but it is nature's way. And nature generally does a darn good job.

She would be surrounded by two or three people she really loves and trusts, with at least one of them trained in childbirth. One of the most important qualities of the professional member of the team is experience, so in a perfect world, this person would have already attended at least a couple hundred births.

The normal birth of a baby is basically a two-step process:

The first portion concerns itself with the dilation of the cervix. Before it begins to open, the cervix is closed tight and resembles perhaps the top of a pop bottle only with the opening more fully closed. During the first part of the labor process, the cervix gradually dilates from tiny opening to ten centimeters of opening, about four inches.

Once this dilation is complete, the second portion kicks into gear. The upper part of the uterus then contracts in such a way that baby is slowly pushed out.

Going back to our ideal delivery, one of the secrets of a lower stress birth is for this portion to progress slowly. The reason for this is if these uterine contractions move slowly, mom's tissues have a chance to gradually change shape to accommodate the stretching and the passage of baby. Baby's head can also change shape temporarily for the passage, and occasionally the bones that make up the top of the skull even fold one over the other briefly. For these reasons, slow is better.

Once baby is out and breathing smoothly, the best place to put the "new arrival" is up on mom's bare chest. Baby might or might not want to nurse, but either way, this is the best place.

The cord should NOT be cut yet. It is important for our baby to gradually supply more and more of his or her own oxygen through breathing, while at the same time decreasing dependency on the oxygen arriving from mom through the umbilical cord.

After a few minutes, the cord will stop pulsating and it should then be tied or clamped. And then it can be cut, about two or three inches out from baby's tummy.

Anything else that anyone was thinking of doing (ointment in eyes, weighing baby) can wait for an hour or two. The only thing that should be done right away is the PKU test, which is accomplished by pricking the heel of the newborn and collecting a tiny droplet of blood.

Ideally, baby has a chance to meet members of the family, look around some and check things out a bit before napping or having anything else done.

While childbirth is natural, that doesn't mean it isn't a lot of work. And yes, it does hurt. In an effort to explain it to a man, one woman said,

"Pinch your upper lip until it hurts and then hold it pinched while pulling this upper lip over the top of your head while running up a mountain for several hours." Probably a pretty good analogy.

There is no "correct" amount of time for the two phases of labor. However, note that the first portion starts slowly and gets harder and harder as mom approaches the 10cm dilation mark. Then, the pushing the baby out phase is generally much harder, but often somewhat faster.

It's important to point out that the pushing referred to here is that which is done by the uterus as it gradually contracts and pushes baby out. I am NOT referring to what you see on TV, where mom is breaking blood vessels in her eyes from straining so hard. In fact, for most deliveries, the best plan is to not push at all (until during the last few contractions when mom cannot help herself no matter what).

OK, that is a quick overview of the process. So now, let's zoom in and take a closer look at some of the pieces.

PART IV

———

KEY DECISIONS
THAT WILL CHANGE
EVERYTHING

Key Decision One:
Selecting A Birth Professional

THIS IS ONE OF YOUR most important decisions because it impacts everything else.

You have two basic choices, physician (obstetrician) and midwife.

Before you get too serious about making any decisions, let's pose some questions so that you can think through who *you* are and how you feel about some of the basics.

- Are you basically strong and healthy?

- If you've already delivered one or more babies, how did things go?

- Are you comfortable in a hospital setting or do hospitals scare you or make you nervous?

- Are you a bit of a contrarian, someone who is comfortable going against the grain?

- Have you primarily heard horror stories about childbirth or have you instead heard tales of positive experiences and pleasant memories?

- Is a birth that is "as natural as possible" one of your goals?

- Are you the type who likes to take control or would you rather someone else ran things?

- Would you like to be involved in all the key decisions related to your delivery?

- Do you believe that delivering a baby is a normal function, one that has been done many millions of times by many millions of women, and one that you too can do?

These questions will help you know who you are, so that you are in a better position to consider the type of delivery you'd like and who should ideally attend the birth.

One deception is seen far too often. It is the physician who says, "Oh yes certainly, I believe in natural birth." But when you look at this doctor's statistics, you'll find 30% cesarean rates, induced labor, pulling on baby's head and all the rest. He just *says* he does things naturally.

I hate to bring money into the equation but statistically, for every $100 more a doctor is paid for a cesarean delivery, the likelihood of cesarean delivery goes up 4%. Hmmm . . .

Also, when you think General Practitioner or Obstetrician, think SURGEON.

So, to get to the truth, you must interview any potential doctor or practitioner. You must also be prepared to walk away and look for another if the one you are interviewing flunks.

How To Interview A Birth Professional

OK, you'll be making a very important decision, so here are some of the most important and enlightening questions to ask when interviewing a potential physician:

- What percentage of the doctor's births are C-section? Hint: if the doctor doesn't know or won't say, he is hiding something.

- After baby is born, how long until the doctor cuts the umbilical cord? The answer you're looking for: "After a few minutes and after the cord has quit pulsing and after baby is breathing great on her own."

- Is the doctor's delivery room usually quiet? Best answer: the doctor likes it quiet, peaceful and even likes to dim the lights as baby arrives.

- How many deliveries has doctor attended? Answer: shoot for a doctor with at least 300 or, hopefully, many more than that.

- What does the doctor say are the pros and cons of using a Midwife to assist with deliveries? Best answer: "They are a great option and I support their use."

- On how many births does this doctor use fetal monitors? Best answer: "We usually don't need them."

- During how much of labor does this doctor think mom should be on her back? And during how much can she be walking around, sitting or squatting? Answer: the more mom is upright and the less she is on her back, the better.

- Will this doctor be available when you go into labor, and what is Plan B if not? There could be several "right" answers here. Make sure *you* are satisfied.

- About how many of this doctor's deliveries are drug induced? Look for a doctor who truthfully can say that not too many are induced.

- Who else does the doctor "approve" to be in delivery room? Regarding this one, see if the answer fits with your goals.

- And the big one (although it's not really a question): are you comfortable and at ease with this doctor?

So again, the professional who'll be attending your birth is a very important first decision. Take your time here and get it right. You'll be so glad you did.

The questions above are given to interview physicians but with slight variations, they can be used to interview most anyone you might be considering attending your birth.

Birth Professional Pros And Cons

Here are a few of the general advantages and disadvantages of each type of birth professional.

Physician/Obstetrician Pros: This professional usually has the highest level of training. If for some reason surgical intervention is needed, it is nice to already be working with a surgeon. This can also be your best choice for a higher risk pregnancy. He or she is there at the hospital every day and knows the area well.

Physician/Obstetrician Cons: My OB friends might get mad for me saying this, but there is some truth in the old saying, "When your only tool is a hammer, everything tends to look like a nail." And while surgery is not their only tool, you would be hard pressed to find many General Practitioners or Obstetricians who can honestly say that the majority of their deliveries were accomplished with no surgical intervention whatsoever.

In contrast, there are many non-MD childbirth professionals who will attend sometimes two or three hundred births in a row with none needing any form of surgical intervention.

Statistically, the difference is too great to be blamed on a run of bad luck or a certain type of mom.

Another issue when considering having an OB as your primary professional is that most all their deliveries are in hospitals. Therefore, if you've had any thoughts about delivering in a birth center or at home, this may not be the choice for you. Also, if the delivery turns into a surgery, all of your personal support group will be asked to leave. One other factor is that an MD/OB is more likely to be male than is a midwife. Just a thought in case this matters much to you.

The last factor is cost. The hospital birth price will total up to between fifteen and forty times as much as one at home or in a birth center with a midwife!

Midwife Pros: With a midwife, there are several possible advantages. Most midwives have a natural philosophy that increases the likelihood of a natural delivery. Almost all are female. Most will assist with your birth in your home or in a birth center, and in many locales, they can attend births at the local hospital too.

Midwives generally have a soothing demeanor coupled with a "can do" attitude. They welcome anyone you would like to have present at your birth and they will usually encourage you to be sitting, squatting or walking about during your labor instead of lying on your back.

Remember that an experienced midwife has successfully attended hundreds of deliveries. Also keep in mind that most deliveries in the history of the world were attended by someone with very little experience or training whatsoever. Compared to this, most midwives are highly trained and experienced.

As mentioned above, provided you are a solid person and are not anticipating a high-risk delivery, it is nice not to have to sell a kidney to pay for a hospital delivery, complete with M.D., anesthesiologist, nurses running in and out and overpriced jello.

Midwife Cons: If you are a genuine high-risk pregnancy, a midwife probably isn't your best option. Some of the high-risk factors include diabetes (temporary gestational or regular), high blood pressure, a non-optimal placenta location, a huge baby in a tiny mom and breech baby position. Some would say that a previous C-section delivery constitutes high risk, but this assertion is generally considered false today.

In addition to the professional(s) at your birth, who else would you like there with you (partner, mom or a girlfriend)? Whatever your answer here, make sure the professional you choose won't fight you and your wishes.

Depending on where you live, there are other options between these two ends of the spectrum such as nurse practitioners and naturopaths. Whatever professional you choose, just make sure you know they are truly on your side and working in accordance with your goals.

Key Decision Two:
Where To Have Your Baby

THIS IS ALSO A BIG item worth careful consideration because it effects the outcome in so many ways.

The overall "feel" of many hospitals is just plain scary, uncomfortable and intimidating. Others feel very homey, with quiet atmospheres and pleasant staff members. Some are more user friendly, encouraging mom to be up and around throughout most of her labor. These same ones are usually very okay with whomever you want there with you.

A birth center may appear to be your best options. But remember, there can be down sides, such as being too far away if surgical intervention is really needed. This can be true of home births also, plus you may have a dog barking or a three-year-old wondering what's going on and all the rest. So really weigh the birth location thoughtfully.

Ok, great! Two big decisions made.

But we're not done with decisions.

Key Decision Three: What Vaccinations WILL You Or WON'T You Allow Them To Give YOU (The Mom)?

MEDICAL WEBSITES PROVIDE a long checklist of substances known to cause birth defects, including acne drugs, some antidepressants and heavy metals such as lead and mercury.

However, when it comes to flu shots (many of which contain mercury), the same website tells women the vaccines are completely safe any time during pregnancy.

But is that true when published reports point to an increased risk of *miscarriages, stillbirth, birth defects and autism* in the offspring of mothers who received influenza vaccines during pregnancy? This has been described by Children's Health Defense on multiple occasions.

Here's another example to watch out for. In 2011, CDC and other medical trade organizations began recommending that all pregnant women get the Tdap triple vaccine (tetanus-diphtheria-acellular pertussis), which, among other ingredients, contains aluminum (known for decades to be a potent neurotoxin and strongly suspected as one of the primary causes of the autism epidemic).

To sort this all out, you just need to remember that whatever is injected into your body during pregnancy will absolutely get into your baby. Please, DO decide and know in advance!

With that, we are now on to the last really big single decision (or it can be a series of individual decisions) you should make long before your baby is born.

Key Decision Four:
What Vaccinations WILL You Or WON'T You Allow Them To Give To Your Baby?

BEFORE DISCUSSING ANY SPECIFIC vaccinations, there is one utmost important truth that needs to be stated.

Vaccination is NOT immunization. Immunization would mean that the shot provides immunity, which is very often not the case. Consider, for instance, the tetanus vaccination. If you were to get a cut or step on a nail, they will almost certainly tell you to get another tetanus shot, even if you've had several tetanus shots before and even if the most recent one was just a couple years back. They have very little confidence in the earlier shots providing immunity.

Also, you should know that large numbers of vaccinated people have been found in all known outbreaks of the diseases for which kids receive vaccinations, and sometimes almost all who got the disease were vaccinated.

Here are some examples.

- Sweden abandoned the whooping cough vaccine due to its ineffectiveness. Out of 5,140 cases in a certain year, it was found that 84% had been vaccinated three times.

- Consider the measles outbreaks that occur with surprising regularity. According to the Journal of the American Medical Association, although more than 95% of school-aged children in the "US" are vaccinated against measles, large measles outbreaks continue to occur in schools, and in most cases, they occur among previously vaccinated children.

- Years ago, Ghana was declared "measles free" by the World Health Organization after 96% of its population was vaccinated. The vaccination program continued, but a mere five years later, Ghana experienced one of the worst measles outbreaks in its history with the highest death rate ever.

- In the United States, mumps is roughly twice as common in vaccinated individuals.

- In the United Kingdom between 1970 and 1990, over 200,000 cases of whooping cough occurred in fully vaccinated children.

It is also often observed that those who get flu shots are more likely to get the flu that year, and often it is within days of the shot. Start asking around. Find someone who got the flu and very likely you're talking to someone who gets flu shots. To dodge the fact that people who get flu shots get the flu, a lame explanation is provided: "They don't get the flu. They just get flu like symptoms (that are exactly like the flu)!"

According to a Canadian study, flu shots cause such severely weakened immunity that death rates go up among those who receive flu shots.

Again, vaccination is NOT immunization. Although health districts, pediatric offices and the CDC have full knowledge of this fact, they still insist on calling all their shots "immunizations." But remember, this itself is just one more act of deception.

BUT . . . what about all the diseases that vaccination eliminated?

You might want to sit down for this: The game-changing, eye-opening fact we are never told is that virtually all the diseases that vaccinations took credit for eradicating were in steep decline *before the vaccination for each disease showed up on the scene.*

Measles is just one of these several diseases that mostly went away before vaccinations, with the death rates decreasing in the United States by 98% before the vaccination was developed.

Almost as dramatic was the decline before vaccinations of typhoid fever, polio, smallpox, diphtheria, yellow fever, tetanus and whooping cough.

In his extremely well documented books, Neil Z. Miller shows how the incidence of (and deaths from) these diseases dropped to near zero before their respective vaccinations came to market. If you have the slightest doubt and want to see proof, I strongly encourage you to order one or all his books.

What is the explanation for this decline before vaccinations? I offer these four possibilities:

- The change was largely due to improved sanitation, less rodents, cleaner water, better food handling and availability of refrigeration.

- The change was partly the result of better heating systems and homes with insulation (versus living in North Dakota with sub-zero winter winds blowing in one side of houses and out the other).

- The diseases to some degree just ran their courses. Keep in mind that the bubonic plague, typhoid, leprosy and the last several ice ages all just went away on their own.

- With some of the diseases, the change was partially due to little things like simply taking baths! Others (tetanus especially) decreased largely due to the population moving off farms where there were more infected rusty nails and into cities where there weren't so many.

I urge you to learn about each disease. Learn about how rare each truly is. Learn how deadly each isn't. Learn what vaccines are used, what is in these vaccines and the dangers posed by these ingredients.

What Vaccinations Will They Try To Give Your Child?

HERE IS A LIST of ALL the vaccinations on the first-24-months schedule *so far*, the ones a pediatrician or children's clinic will attempt to give your baby before his or her second birthday unless you stop this from happening:

1. Hepatitis B vaccination at birth

2. Another Hepatitis B vaccination at one to two months

3. Diphtheria vaccination at two months

4. Tetanus vaccination at two months

5. Pertussis vaccination at two months

6. Haemophilus influenza type B vaccination at two months

7. Poliovirus vaccination at two months

8. Pneumococcal conjugate vaccination at two months

9. Rotavirus vaccination at two months

10. Diphtheria vaccination at four months

11. Tetanus vaccination at four months

12. Pertussis vaccination at four months

13. Haemophilus influenza type B vaccination at four months

14. Poliovirus vaccination at four months

15. Pneumococcal conjugate vaccination at four months

16. Rotavirus vaccination at four months

17. Diphtheria vaccination at six months

18. Tetanus vaccination at six months

19. Pertussis vaccination at six months

20. Haemophilus influenza type B vaccination at six months

21. Pneumococcal conjugate vaccination at six months

22. Rotavirus vaccination at six months

23. Influenza (Flu) vaccination at about one year

24. Hepatitis B vaccination at about one year

25. Polio Virus Vaccination at about one year

26. Hepatitis A vaccination at about one year

27. Haemophilus influenza type B vaccination at about one year

28. Measles vaccination at about 16 months

29. Mumps vaccination at about 16 months

30. Rubella vaccination at about 16 months

31. Pneumococcal conjugate vaccination at about 16 months

32. Chickenpox vaccination at about 22 months

33. Influenza (Flu) vaccination at about 22 months

34. Hepatitis A vaccination at about 22 months

35. Diphtheria vaccination at 22 months

36. Tetanus vaccination at 22 months

37. Pertussis vaccination at 22 months

O U C H ! ! ! That's 37 vaccinations by age two.

Scary? It gets worse. Below is a partial list of ingredients found in these 37 vaccinations they want to give your baby before age two:

- Aluminium: attacks central nervous system and results in brain damage. Each time vaccinations are given to babies, they receive 30 to 40 times as much aluminum as the FDA says is safe. (FDA looks the other way when it comes to vaccinations.)

- Amphotericin B: potentially fatal cardiac or cardiopulmonary arrest.

- Formaldehyde: embalming fluid, known cause of cancer and to damage nerves, liver and kidneys.

- Thimerosal (this is half mercury): mercury is one of the most neurotoxic substances on earth. There is no safe level of exposure, especially in babies.

- 2-Phenoxyethanol: may cause chromosomal changes, genetic mutations, testicular atrophy, shock, convulsions, cardiac failure and death.

- Glutaraldehyde: causes asthma, allergic reactions, respiratory trouble and diarrhea.

- Sodium taurodeoxycholate: a detergent! May break down blood-brain barrier, allowing dangerous toxins into the brain.

- Casein (from cows): may cause severe allergic reactions.

- Chlortetracyclin: an antibiotic. May disrupt healthy bacteria cultures and harm immunity.

- Ovalbumin (from chicken eggs): causes allergic reactions, especially inflammation of the air passageways in lungs and bronchial tubes.

- Gelatin (from pigs): can cause anaphylactic shock reactions.

- Gentamicin Sulfate: this antibiotic can cause allergic reactions.

- Latex (like in rubber gloves): causes allergic reactions.

- Neomycin (an antibiotic): may cause local or whole-body allergic reactions.

- Polymyxin B: results in toxicity and severe pain or inflammation at injection site.

- Serum (from baby calves): inhumanely harvested, with small risk of contamination.

- Streptomycin: an antibiotic. A baby may be severely allergic to it.

- Yeast: may cause autoimmune disease.

- MF59: linked to autoimmunity and chronic disease.

- Human serum albumin: taken from aborted fetuses.

- Recombinant albumin: may cause baby's immune system to attack and damage his own body.

- Sorbitol: increases the risk of diabetes and cell death.

- Emulsifiers: may cause inflammatory bowel disease.

- Yeast: can cause headaches, sleeping disorders, irritable bowel, asthma, diabetes, seizures and shock.

- Genetically modified organisms: no one knows what these may cause because no tests have been done.

Considering a baby is designed to *only* have breast milk before age two months, how severely shocked is baby when all this garbage is injected? And how will baby's very immature immune system revolt and react?

Babies simply aren't ready to ride bulls in the rodeo, smoke cigars, drink whiskey or get vaccinations.

How Vaccinations Prevent Health

Isn't HEALTH THE GOAL? If so, wouldn't it make sense to compare the health of vaccinated kids against unvaccinated kids? Well, our medical system went on and on for decades, adding one vaccination after another to the schedule. Shown below is a compilation of data from various sources which finally compares vaccinated against unvaccinated.

Unvaccinated children were found to be healthier in virtually every way.

Vaccinated kids are:

- Twice as likely to have asthma

- 30 times as likely to have hay fever

- 11 times as likely to have epilepsy

- 5 times as likely to have learning disabilities

- 7 times as likely to have tubes put in their ears

- 3 times as likely to have middle ear infections

- 22 times as likely to use allergy medication

- 6 times as likely to get pneumonia

- 3 times as likely to have chronic disease

- 4 times as likely to have tonsillitis

- twice as likely to have ulcerative colitis

- 3 times as likely to have Crohn's disease

- dozens of times as likely to have autism

Also, vaccinated babies are more likely to die in their sleep. And after vaccinations, children are significantly more prone to later have diabetes, measles, mumps and even cancer.

There may have been other variables which were not put into the equation, and again, the only factor considered was simply whether they were vaccinated or not.

Now we have been told for decades that vaccinations are safe and effective. Every time I heard that, I would get this nagging deja vu feeling. It always reminded me of something else, a different situation but the same story. Finally it came to me!

For 40 years, hormone replacement therapy was prescribed for most women during and after menopause. After about 20 years of this, the drug companies decided they wanted to *sell even more* of these hormones. They began telling physicians that their female patients should stay on these hormones *for life* because the drugs lowered each woman's risk of heart disease, stroke and osteoporosis. Finally, after a full 40 years, a proper, long-term study was begun to assess the real risks versus any supposed benefits. The plan was for this study to go on for at least ten years. However, *within months, the risk of increased heart disease, stroke, blood clots and breast cancer were so obvious the study was shut down years early!*

I am absolutely certain that if a real, untainted, long-term study compared the health of vaccinated versus unvaccinated children, the difference would be just as glaring. But who will do the study? Not the CDC, FDA, pediatricians or pharmaceutical companies, you can be confident of that. The money from vaccination is simply to much to give up.

Few people realize that vaccines have also been linked to brain damage, lowered IQ, learning disabilities, ADHD and brain dysfunction, even though all this is well known among legitimate researchers. In fact, neurological disorders are among the most listed and studied vaccine complications in the medical literature.

Here is what I am asserting: vaccinations cause more diseases than they prevent and are not safe or effective despite what we are told. They are one of the major reasons thirty-two million American children, 43% of the total number, suffer from at least one of 20 chronic illnesses, and many of these same children have two or more.

Yes, vaccinations are playing a major role in this onslaught of disease. Compared to their parents, children today are *four times* more likely to develop a chronic illness.

Many of the vaccinations are for conditions your child cannot realistically get, such as diphtheria and polio. Diphtheria simply isn't around where we live, and it is a long-acknowledged fact that all cases of polio in North America since 1947 were caused by the polio vaccine!

Many other vaccinations are given for conditions you want your child to get. Chicken pox, flu, measles and mumps are examples. Why get these perfectly normal childhood diseases? First, children get *real* and usually *lifelong* immunity. Second, getting *more* fever-causing diseases when young translates to *less* cancer when older (but don't hold your breath waiting for the American Cancer Society to mention that fact). And third, a mom-to-be who got these conditions naturally when she was young passes this immunity on to her baby, where it will usually last through the first couple years of life.

Here's another important point: no one on earth has any idea whether your child is allergic to any of the ingredients until *after* there is an adverse reaction. Your baby may get five, six or even seven vaccinations in a single visit to a doctor, but no tests have ever been done to determine whether multiple shots given at one time is safe. What about cumulative poisoning from vaccine ingredients? Has that been studied? No, not even aluminum, which may surpass safe limits *forty fold* on each "well baby" visit.

Even when individual vaccines are tested, the test subjects are just followed for a few days or perhaps for a couple of weeks. Is that really long enough, considering many of the worst effects don't show up for months or even years?

As an example, formaldehyde is a known cause of cancer. But cancer certainly isn't going to appear during the four days after vaccination. (Four days is the length of time babies were formally observed following injection with each of several formaldehyde-laced vaccines.) Is four days really long enough? Consider the fact that when formaldehyde was diluted with water to make it one-fifth as concentrated as what is in dozens of childhood vaccines, it frequently caused cancer at that level when injected into animals.

Some babies scream inconsolably for hours, even *days* after vaccination, indicating swelling of their brains. Some get lumps at the injection site or a huge, swollen leg on that side. Some clearly regress into autism almost immediately. Many have other serious vaccine injuries. Tragically, some babies even die shortly after being vaccinated.

In spite of all this, physicians are very hesitant to lay the blame on the obvious culprit. Even when their babies go into convulsions or became paralyzed within hours of after vaccination, parents are still told, "It was just a coincidence." Doctors don't want word to get out that a baby reacted violently or died after a visit to their office. And they don't want to be sued.

Medical publications regularly tell us that a tiny few out of the total are reported!

Some vaccinations are given at the wrong time in the child's life, so that any immunity derived is gone before it is needed. The dangers from the vaccine may greatly overshadow any benefits. Again, a perfect example of this is the tetanus vaccination. They will try to give your baby three shots of it before baby is even crawling. What are the possibilities of this baby getting a deep puncture wound from a rusty barnyard nail at that age?

After all these toxin-ladened tetanus shots, we discover that the chances of anyone under age 50 dying from tetanus today are less than one in one billion (this is the actual calculation)!

By the way, I urge you to stay away from the promotional materials put out by the pharmaceutical companies that are making billions of dollars from these vaccinations. Put aside any ideas you may have that they are telling the truth. Unload any opinions you may already have formed that are based on their propaganda. Take a fresh, unbiased look. Then, really think about whether all (or any) of these vaccinations are truly needed by your child.

As stated above, it is IMPERATIVE that you make decisions regarding the vaccinations long before a nurse or doctor is walking toward your baby with a syringe in hand. (I did exactly this. Because of the decisions made, if you add together all my children, you'll find that they combined are more than 700 vaccinations behind schedule, which cost the entire vaccination business around $40,000! Whoops!)

A final note on vaccinations: The National Vaccination Injury Compensation Program has paid out over $3,700,000,000,000 to vaccination injured children and the families of those who were killed by "perfectly safe" vaccinations. Although a CDC funded study found that less than 1% of vaccination injuries were reported, that 1% amounted to hundreds of thousands of claims being filed for vaccine injury, of which over 88,000 were awarded compensation so far. And get this: *to even be considered for this compensation, damage from the vaccination must show up within days.* In view of the fact that the vast majority of vaccination damage shows up much, much later, can you imagine the number of families who experience vaccine injury but will never qualify for this compensation?

I'm simply saying there are *millions* of vaccine injuries. Most *appear* to be small, but even with these, we will never know how much better, how much more alive, any given child could have been without this damage. Small amounts of damage to a child's immunity, to his mental ability, to his genetic code (DNA), these are not small things.

Remember many vaccine injuries are severe. Some are absolutely deadly. And about all of them are permanent.

Can The Vaccination Program Be Made Safer?

WHAT WOULD IT TAKE to make vaccination safer?

This is a very valid question, but one which I will have to somewhat force myself to answer. After we've all been deceived dozens of ways and outright lied to for decades regarding vaccinations, I'm a bit sore about the whole topic.

But okay, I'll try to be nice! Here are some actions that would make vaccinations much safer:

First, remove the most toxic elements and chemicals from vaccines and replace them with safer ones. Thimerosal (half mercury) and formaldehyde (embalming fluid) are examples of these toxic ingredients. Thimerosal is already out of some vaccinations - after years of public outcry. But even now, it still remains in roughly 30% of the vaccine doses children receive depending on the clinic and the region. Safer alternatives could no doubt be found for most of the more dangerous and toxic ingredients.

Second, eliminate the vaccinations for the childhood diseases that are both beneficial and relatively harmless. Chickenpox would certainly be included on this list. But despite all the noise to the contrary, so could measles, mumps, rubella, rubeola and Hepatitis B.

Third, eliminate those vaccinations for diseases that are almost impossible to die from today in our modern country. These would include, among others, tetanus, diphtheria, smallpox and polio.

Fourth, get rid of all combination vaccines such as DPT (diphtheria, pertussis, and tetanus) and MMR (measles, mumps, or rubella). Break them up into single vaccines and give them on separate days.

And fifth, after all the above is done, give any remaining vaccinations when children are a year or two older. The immune system of a baby is absolutely not mature enough to handle the assault of vaccination. As an example mentioned elsewhere in this book, when just one shot was postponed for two years in Japan, the crib death rates fell immediately.

Well there, I gave "how to improve vaccination safety" a shot! But truth is, no matter what changes are made, there are a number of areas where vaccinations will still be problematic. As just one of many examples, childhood diseases such as measles and mumps were rarely harmful when they occurred naturally at the ages when they naturally occurred, usually around ages four, five or six. However, vaccinating for these two conditions caused a chain of events that ended with *newborns* and *adults* getting measles and mumps instead. And at these ages, both are somewhat dangerous. Can this be undone? Yes. But it would take probably fifty years with no vaccinations given for either.

The Great Flu Shot Hoax

BEFORE MOVING ON, I want to give you a bit of behind the scenes viewing of one of the common vaccinations, the infamous flu shot. Among many big frauds, flu shots are one of the biggest. Let's take a close look.

There are thousands of strains of influenza and new ones appearing every day. In spite of this, we are supposed to believe the geniuses at the drug companies can guess which variation is going to be the "big one" next winter and develop a shot for that mutation before it exists anywhere on the planet. Amazing!

As the "flu season" approaches each year, there is media frenzy about how deadly the flu will be. And worse (according to the sources for this media frenzy), there will be a shortage of flu vaccinations. Terrible!

One early media blast a couple years ago (radio, TV, newspapers, the works) told how five seniors had died in one county alone. I picked up the phone and called the health department of that county and asked about it. The officer replied, "Actually, the flu was a contributing factor in all five deaths, but these were very old people. Each had several serious conditions and none were expected to live very long with or without the flu. *And they all were fully vaccinated for the flu!*"

What happened to the great "flu epidemic" that year? Less than 400 people in the U. S. died, about one out of every million Americans. And then, after scaring the country half to death and selling every last shot, the perpetrators later admitted that the vaccination they had sold wasn't even close to the right shot for the flu strain they had said would be so deadly. Maybe I missed it but I don't remember them giving back the two billion dollars they conned out of the public for this fiasco.

Here's a humorous postscript to this. The next winter, a doctor was accused and charged for injecting leftover shots from that year into people the next year. His "crime" was giving patients the wrong shot for that season's flu, which was exactly what *all* doctors had done the winter before!

In case you're curious how they decide what vaccine they will make and which strain of flu it will address, *per their materials* here's how it is done: an FDA advisory panel selects three flu strains it believes will be circulating in the coming season. (This represents very skilled use of a crystal ball.) Once selected, a statement is virtually always made that goes like this: "The flu strain expected this year is known to cause more hospitalizations than other strains." (To achieve this level of detail and accuracy, an Ouija board was also employed.)

OK, that's what they tell us. However, if the promoters of the flu vaccines were interested in telling the truth, a typical year's press releases would read more like this: "Last flu season, 65% of Americans did not get flu shots. Even among the chronically ill, barely half got flu shots. Of infants in the (supposedly) high risk 6 month to two-year age group, only 22% got flu shots. Despite a dismally poor showing for the shots, and even in the face of a predicted 'deadly' strain, there were only a few hundred deaths."

Dr. J. Anthony Morris (former Chief Vaccine Control Officer at the U.S. Federal Drug Administration), has this to say: "There is no evidence that any influenza vaccine thus far developed is effective in preventing or mitigating any attack of influenza. The producers of these vaccines know that they are worthless, but they go on selling them anyway." Please, read that statement again and note again who made it.

You've surely observed this for yourself. Think of each person you know who really got sick with the flu. Yep, most of them had received a flu shot!

I saw this too. Years ago, I knew several students who attended a certain private college. The entire student body got flu shots and they pretty much had to close down the school for the next week and a half. *Everyone* got the flu. After observing this occurring time and time again over the years, I don't personally believe that flu shots decrease flu or flu deaths. If anything, I would be more inclined to believe that flu shots actually increase the incidence of flu.

All that said, I just have these few last words specifically about infant flu shots, and THIS IS IMPORTANT: *over 90% of the individuals on the board that recommended infant flu shots have financial interests in vaccine manufacture and distribution.*

And that explains about everything!

Well OK, let's leave the topic of vaccinations for the moment and back up a few months. Let's get to working on things you should do for a healthy pregnancy. The factors here are much like they would be at any stage of a person's life: diet, exercise, sleep, attitude, attempting to not gain 100 pounds, etc. But what you do with each of these factors when you're pregnant can be considerably different.

PART V

———

THE HEALTHY
PREGNANCY

Twenty-Second Chapter

Supplementation During Pregnancy

IN A PAGE OR TWO, we'll get into what you will want to be eating through your pregnancy. But in this little section, we'll discuss the added supplementation that is smart to add to your diet:

Folic Acid: folic acid is a B Vitamin that everyone needs. But you should have more during pregnancy because developing babies really need it. You can get it from various fresh vegetables including leafy salad-type vegetables, so eat plenty. Best still to supplement. Ask for "Folate." It's the best form of this vitamin.

Iron: more iron is needed during pregnancy for the extra blood that your body will produce. But remember, iron from the wrong sources will plug you up, and constipation during pregnancy isn't all that fun.

Calcium: a developing baby will use quite a bit of calcium. If you don't have extra in your diet, baby will take it from your bones and teeth. Again, the source of this calcium is important. (I'll get to that part soon.)

Vitamin D: this vitamin comes from sunlight. If you live where it is sunny, go out in the sun and you'll get plenty. In low sun areas (or low sun seasons), you should supplement.

DHA: DHA is one of the valuable nutritional oils commonly found in quality fish. Make sure the fish you eat (or fish oil) isn't farmed. Farmed fish is far worse than none at all (unless you are starving). Nut oils are exceptionally good.

Iodine: while this is an important element in your pregnancy diet, simply continuing with iodized salt should meet your needs.

Nutrition During Pregnancy

THE BEST NUTRITION (including vitamins and minerals) always comes from real food sources. With that in mind, let me here include a quick review of how things are designed in nature to work.

The first and biggest concept is this: plants "eat" minerals. We then eat the plants, or we eat something that ate the plants. We do not get our minerals directly from rock or out of the ground. You can't get iron from sucking on a rusty nail or calcium from eating chalk. Minerals need to first be converted by plants.

Similarly, the best vitamins by far are those from plant sources.

Next time you are in a grocery store, purposely go down the "don't ever" aisles and look at the "liquid meal" products for adults (Ensure, for instance) and those for babies (like Enfamil or Similac). Read the labels and you will see all the inorganic minerals (they've never been in a plant) and synthetic vitamins (made in a laboratory).

So that's the first thing, understanding the difference between plant based and everything else.

Next, ever hear of a pregnant woman having cravings for odd foods like pistachio ice cream or sour pickles? What this means is that she has nutritional deficiencies. Remember that when this occurs, she is looking for more of *something*. And that *real* something she's craving isn't likely to be ice cream or pizza. It is something that is found in real food!

OK, so what should she do to handle these cravings?

The best bet, if available, is a broad variety of organic foods. Organic foods are different in that they are grown without poisons, grown in real soil and they are non-GMO (not genetically modified).

I went into a lot of food detail in Chapter 6, but I'll quickly state again some of the advantages of organic foods. They are generally grown by people who know that plants grown on rich, healthy soil are naturally full of the nutrients we need. These farmers consciously avoid poisonous pesticides, chemical weed killers and artificial fertilizers. They are paid for their products based on true quality, not just quantity. They don't use GMO seeds because they know that no long-term studies have been done on what harm genetically modified foods may do to humans and because they know that poisons are built right into GMO crops that in turn pass directly into you. That is why organic is much better whenever possible.

Sugar and chemical sweeteners should be avoided. Again, I could go into quite a bit of detail here, but you have a computer and the internet. Search "safe, healthy sweeteners" to learn about great products like stevia and coconut nectar .

Similarly, starches should largely be avoided, and certainly the commercial ones that don't specify that they are organic. There are two reasons: first, all the commercially grown wheat, rice, corn and potatoes are either GMO or are grown in super-poisoned dirt. Second, you probably don't really want to gain 120 pounds. So, avoid sugars and starches as much as possible while pregnant.

Great food choices during your pregnancy include organic vegetables, beans, seeds and nuts. Organic eggs are exceptional, and you can eat as many as you want. (I will fill you in on the "cholesterol myth" sometime soon.) Organically grown beef and chicken are great (unless you're vegetarian, of course), and wild grown fish such as salmon and halibut are hard to beat.

Avoid all chemical beverages. And don't forget to drink lots of water.

A quick note that I don't want to forget because this is something that could possibly occur: IF in late pregnancy you develop high blood pressure (which may be named preeclampsia or toxemia), the smart solution is to significantly increase your protein intake quickly. This can be done through consuming high protein foods such as eggs, meat and cottage cheese. If this is in fact the correct solution (and it usually is), your blood pressure will be back down in just a couple days. It's very effective.

Germs, Sleep, Stretch Marks, Exercise And Comfort

ONE OF THE BEST exercises is walking, lots of walking. And this should include plenty of walking up hills or stairs. Treadmills and elliptical exercisers are great too. If available, attend a low impact aerobics class. The idea is, you want to keep moving, keep the fluids flowing and keep your heart and lungs in great shape.

Swimming is an excellent exercise, but avoid chlorinated pools if possible.

To get comfortable during pregnancy, many women like to sit on a pillow on the floor with their legs crossed in front of them. An added advantage of this is that it helps to stretch some of the parts that will need to be more limber during the birth process.

Another winning position is to get into a knee chest position by getting on hands and knees and letting your tummy relax down or by putting your head, neck and chest on a couch with your knees on the floor, again letting your tummy sag toward the floor.

Massage is great throughout your pregnancy, with some massage practitioners specially trained in pregnancy massage.

Chiropractic is also a very smart thing to include in your pregnancy.

There are several reasons why, but the most important are a) to keep your nervous system functioning at its best, b) to make sure your pelvis isn't twisted (because that can make your delivery difficult), c) for your comfort and d) to be around yet another supportive natural-thinking person.

Stretch Mark Avoidance Tip

You are going to do some serious growing, both in your tummy and in your breasts. If you are interested in reducing stretch marks, it is smart to start early with applications of a good natural oil such as that from avocado, coconut or almond. Do a quick internet search regarding locations where stretch marks may occur so you know where to focus your efforts.

Better Sleep During Pregnancy

Make sure you get lots of sleep. It doesn't have to all be at night either. Naps are good! Also, as you get very near the end of your pregnancy, make sure you stay rested at all times because, once labor starts, you're going to need some serious energy.

As the months of your pregnancy advance, sleeping can become quite an ordeal. Starting in your 7th or 8th month, you may want to keep about five pillows near your bed. As you prepare to lay on your side, put one between your ankles and another between your knees. Put one or two under the baby section (so that your spine is less twisted). Finally, the last pillow goes under your head.

A Note on Germs

The use of antiseptic soaps and disinfectants kills roughly 99.9% of germs, and that is exactly why they are dangerous. The tough microbes that aren't killed are the ones that repopulate the earth. Therefore, every time someone uses one of these products, they are contributing to the creation of super germs that will be difficult if not impossible to kill down the road. Also remember that most bacteria are beneficial and therefore, you don't want to kill them. Blasting bacteria with antibiotics and hand sanitizer is like bombing a town to get rid of a few criminals.

Baby's Position Before Going Into Labor

If the professional who will be attending your birth is good, he or she should be able to tell if your baby is positioned correctly for the easiest birth. If it is found that baby is not in the ideal head down, face backward position, baby can most always be turned. This process requires the use of an ultrasound and a doctor who knows what to do. Most major cities have a few such individuals who specialize in turning babies, and they are worth seeking out if baby would otherwise be presenting wrong.

A Note Regarding Dry Cleaning

The chemicals tatrachloroethylene and perchloroethylene (big words, poisonous chemicals) are the most commonly used dry cleaning solvents. They are known to cause umbilical cord deformities and miscarriage, and are therefore well worth avoiding.

Decide NOW What How Things Are Going To Be After Baby Is Born

It is smart to have things all worked out so that after baby is born, you will have a couple days of serenity and peace to recover and get to know your baby. It's also good to know in advance who you will want to notify first with the news and to have a list so you don't forget anyone who would be hurt if they weren't told.

There are so many questions that may arise. Therefore, I encourage you to become part of our private "Smart Parent Inner Circle" Facebook group, where you can ask questions of like-minded people. Not only will you get their support, but I'll also be there several times most every day of the year to answer questions and offer suggestions. (Go to SmartMomHealthyBaby in Facebook to learn more.)

OK, you're getting very close to delivery time. You've made several important decisions. You know where you will be having the baby, what professional will be attending to the birth and who else you have invited to join you.

PART VI

———

THE LOW STRESS
DELIVERY

Summary Of What Makes
A Most Ideal Delivery

- You're all set in advance to have baby in a "safe" location where you won't be pressured, distracted or bullied.

- You have it worked out so you will be attended by professionals and/or others who are very supportive of YOUR choices.

- You are well fed (but with no food during the last hours before delivery), in pretty good shape and have had plenty of sleep.

- Baby is pointed the right direction: head down and facing backwards.

- You know who will be in the birth room with you and who won't.

- Everyone is to be quiet as baby arrives, with the lights dimmed right at birth if possible.

- You know how you will be spending most of labor: walking around, sitting and squatting ideally, and not on your back.

- You've already decided what anesthetic and surgical procedures (including C-section) you will or won't allow and under what circumstances.

- You have given specific instructions on who holds the baby right after delivery (ideally you and your partner) and what baby can be fed (nursing is best).

This Is How Labor Starts

DURING THE LAST COUPLE months of pregnancy, it is common to have light contractions called Braxton Hicks contractions. These are basically warm up, practice contractions to get you in shape for the real thing.

Real labor is different in that the contractions are frequent and regular. Initially, "frequent" may be every ten minutes. And regular might not be all that regular.

Gradually, the contractions do become regular and more intense. By the time they are at about four minutes apart and consistent, you'll want to be getting close to wherever you intend to have your baby.

At some point in the process, your amniotic sac will usually burst (your water will break). If it breaks *before* labor starts, you will need to deliver in the hospital. Occasionally the membrane will hold tough and not break until after the cervix is dilated and baby is on his way out. But usually it happens while you're sitting in church, at a graduation or in a banquet. Gives you a better story to tell later. OK, just joking. It breaks *somewhere*. You're probably at home making dinner in your kitchen.

IF your choice is to have your baby at the hospital and IF you have any doubts about willingness of the hospital staff to cooperate with your plans for minimal medical intervention, the next chapter offers some suggestions that may reduce your risk.

Key Times When It Is Smart To Wait

Wait To Go TO The Hospital

Talk this over with your practitioner. Generally speaking, you're waiting for steady, frequent contractions. When your contractions are regular and strong, and coming every four to five minutes for one to two hours, you should be getting with your midwife or doctor soon. A contraction is considered strong if it's difficult to talk through it.

Wait To Go INTO The Hospital

If you get to the hospital and contractions aren't too hard or heavy, it's not a bad idea to stay outside and relax in the car or walk around. It's smart to have all hospital papers filled out before arrival. Or you can go into the hospital but just wait around in some common area such as the lobby or the lunch room. Generally, the sooner you come under the hospital's jurisdiction, the more they will feel the need to earn their money and therefore *do things*, most of which you may not really want.

Wait To Be Placed On Your Back

Sure, for doctors or nurses to check you (dilation, etc.), you may need to get on your back briefly. Other than that, stay upright and moving as long as possible. When it finally is time to lay back during the last contractions (or pushes) of your delivery, it is excellent to assume a semi-supine position (halfway between sitting and laying on your back, your whole trunk and head resting on a huge wedge). Other than for these and a few other less common reasons, sitting, squatting and walking are far better than lying on your back. (Note: this was said before but it bears repeating: when you are on your back late in pregnancy or during delivery, the blood supply to baby is choked off by baby's weight and really ups the stress factor. Try to avoid this.)

Wait To Push

Yep, I really said that! Despite all the blood vessel popping straining you see in the shows, here's what is better: you want to fight the urge to push as long as possible. This is one of the primary reasons for doing the "panting" breathing exercise with each contraction, sort of a distraction tactic.

There are two main reasons to fight the pushing urge as long as possible. As mentioned before, the first is that the more slowly the baby comes out, the more that your tissues will have time to slowly give, stretch and release, thus reducing mom's exposure to tearing and damage. The second reason is that the bones on top of baby's head can temporarily partially fold over one another. Remember, a human head is made of 22 bones, with the upper portion comprised of half a dozen. These bones aren't fused together and can temporarily shift as much as perhaps half an inch if the labor moves slowly enough. Then, not long after baby is out, the plates of the head return to their normal places.

NOTE: there are certain emergency situations where you must push fast and hard. If your practitioner says you have one of these and need to push, do so with all your might.

Wait To Hook Up A Fetal Monitor

Fetal monitors can detect distress in the baby. However, to put one to use, the mom-to-be is almost always placed on her back which, unfortunately, virtually always causes the fetal distress that the monitor is then going to detect! In my opinion, harmful fetal stress is decreased 90% by simply keeping mom off her back. How long should one wait to get hooked up? Well, I'd say most of the time, monitors are totally unnecessary and cause undo worrying over nothing. In general, it's better to just quit causing the stress. However, you picked this practitioner and need to trust him or her. Hopefully they won't put you on your back prematurely to use a fetal monitor without some real and legitimate reason.

Wait (Forever) To Pull On Baby's Head

Babies' heads and necks have for decades been damaged by physicians pulling on them during delivery. The most brutal example was found with the use of forceps, with hundreds of thousands of babies seriously damaged and millions mildly to moderately damaged (faces and heads smashed so they were very asymmetrical, for instance).

More recently, vacuum extractors have become popular (they work like a toilet plunger). They can cause anything from mild bruising to severe, life-threatening damage.

It is far better to let mom's uterus push and gravity assist. But don't be totally against a vacuum assist. If there is legitimate fetal distress (that's not being caused by some sort of stupidity) and the goal is to get baby out fast without a cesarean, the vacuum assist is one of the better options.

The ideal delivery, remember, is where the practitioner either does nothing other than report progress and gently guides baby's journey until it's time to catch the slippery little guy. By the way, after the head is out, the shoulders can follow with greater ease if baby turns sideways.

Wait To Cut The Umbilical Cord

As mentioned earlier, this was a classic blunder for decades. Before babies had a chance to start breathing on their own, rush-job physicians would cut baby's umbilical cords. The result was much like netting a fish and dumping it on the dock, totally and suddenly cutting off its source of oxygen. So know well that your baby should be breathing smoothly, and the umbilical cord should have quit pulsating first. *Then* it is safe to tie off and cut the umbilical cord.

Wait To Put Drops / Ointment Into Baby's Eyes

While putting some antibiotic solution is a smart precaution (and in some cases even prevents blindness), it doesn't need to be done right away. Why not let baby look around a bit, see who is there and make a couple friends before gooping up his or her eyes?

Wait To Separate Baby From Mom (And Dad If He's There)

The best place for baby during the first minutes after birth as mentioned earlier is against mom's bare skin, usually her chest and ideally nursing a bit. This is an excellent bonding time plus it helps the uterus contract into a tight ball and stop any bleeding that was continuing. And don't let anyone put the little, wet baby on a cold, hard scale. There are warmer ways to weigh a baby!

Well, that sums up most of the pregnancy and delivery information, and more specifically, what you need to know and pre-decide to have a low stress pregnancy and delivery.

But there is much more you'll need to know for your baby to continue to be healthy. Once again, this has more to do with what to avoid than what to do.

I've mentioned the high incidence of asthma, allergies, autism, ADHD, cancer, obesity and diabetes several times. So rather than going into a lot of detail with what you should do, let's look at each of these conditions one by one so you know what to avoid. We'll explore the one thing that neither the associations nor your practitioner will likely mention about each of these conditions, what CAUSES them.

PART VII

HOW CHILDREN CAN AVOID THE MOST DANGEROUS CONDITIONS

Vertebral Subluxation And Pressure On Spinal Nerves

WHEN I WAS 5 years old, I was involved in a car accident, which, it turned out, changed the entire course of my life.

I was just a little kid, it was summertime, and I was walking beside the country road in front of our house. The sun setting directly up the road to the west.

A car was also traveling west on that same stretch of road at the very same time. Unfortunately, the sun momentarily blinded the driver of this car. Suddenly he heard a thump-bump at the front of the car. He knew he had hit something, and when he stopped and got out of the car, he found that he had hit ME. I was now laying lifelessly in the ditch.

I found out later that the bumper had struck me in the back of my pelvis, the hood had hit my head, and I was knocked out ... for over 20 minutes.

I was rushed to the emergency room. The doctor there listened to my heart, looked in my eyes and felt the bump on my head. Finally, he stood up and announced, "He'll be OK."

But ... the doctor was wrong. I wasn't OK. The very next day, my left leg started aching, like a terrible toothache. Back to the doctor we went, but all he could say was that I had "growing pains." Of course, even then, I was wondering why this thing he called "growing pains" had come on so suddenly, why was it only in my one leg and why my brother (growing twice as fast) didn't have them. Anyhow, nothing was done for me.

I gradually developed a number of other problems that seemed to be unrelated, including nervousness. Other kids in school would make fun of me because my face twitched. I also got side aches when I ran and a weird tickle in my throat that made me always cough. I even started having acid burning in my stomach.

I was given drugs for these problems, but you have to ask yourself: was there anything wrong with me that drugs could *really* help? Were any of my troubles caused by a lack of drugs?

The months turned into years, and all these problems persisted. I even started having trouble sleeping such that I would lay awake at night, just couldn't fall asleep, usually until around 3:00 A.M. Then, I was so groggy every day in school that I'd fall asleep and get bad grades.

I was taken to doctors again and again, but none of them could ever figure out what was causing a single one of my problems. I just kept getting worse.

During summer vacation after my seventh grade, yet another problem surfaced. I was walking past my older brother in a pair of cutoff shorts when he said, "Look at your leg! It's shrunken."

And he was right! There it was. My left leg was far smaller around than my right leg. It looked like I'd had polio or something and I thought, "How can this be? How could my leg get like this, and without any of us noticing?"

We went to the doctors again. They all looked at my shrunken leg, but all they could say was, "You've grown that way and you're stuck with it. Get used to it." And you know, we all do find ourselves learning to live with things, don't we. We gradually get used to pains and problems, and maybe even get to a point where we don't notice them all that much.

That's what the doctors wanted me to do. They told me to learn to live with it. They didn't have any way to help me, and I realized, "What other choice did I have but to put up with my shrunken leg?"

Summer went on and soon it was July. I started getting jobs with farmers, helping them bring hay in from their fields.

One day, about three weeks into the haying season, I was throwing a bale up onto the trailer as I had by now done several hundred times. But *this* time was different. Something suddenly shifted in my neck, and I got this extreme, intense pain. My neck hurt like I was being stabbed with a knife. My head was pulled uncontrollably to the side, pinning my right ear to my right shoulder, and I couldn't move it. I was stuck like that.

I remember the farmer and his wife standing me up and taking a look at me. "Looks like he has something wrong with his neck, Gertie. What do you think?"

I was obviously done throwing bales for the day, so the farmer took me home. I remember hurrying straight to the mirror to see what was going on, and my heart just sank. School was starting in a few weeks. I'd already been teased so much last year by the other kids because of the nervous twitches and sleeping in class. Now was I going to have to face them like this, looking totally deformed?

Well, as you can imagine, by now we were losing confidence in ordinary doctors. In fact, I wondered why we even bothered with them. But . . . we headed into town one more time to see what the family physician would say about my neck.

The doctor checked me out briefly, and said that I had a "muscle spasm." He wanted to give me a "shot" in the "spasm" side and also put me in a neck brace. But . . . somehow . . . my parents just didn't feel like this was the right answer, so . . . they thanked the doctor and *for the first time ever,* we got up and . . . *we left!*

Now my mom had heard about a doctor . . . a totally different type of doctor, one who worked only with the spine and nerve system. My parents decided that it won't hurt to check him out and see what he would say. We were able to get an appointment that evening and soon were there in his office.

Dr. King asked me some questions. And he examined me, but it wasn't one bit like how I had always been examined before. He was far more thorough, and he focused mostly on my back and my totally-out-of-control neck.

Finally he said, "Look, here's the situation. You have something called "vertebral subluxation." He went on to tell me, "A subluxation is where a vertebra gets out of place and partially paralyzes some of your nerves. That's your problem." He explained that this vertebra could be put back into place and that it would help me.

We thought, "Well, this is different!" We were accustomed to drugs and surgery being about the only treatments that were used for anything. Maybe that's been your experience too.

He analyzed me a little more and explained what he was going to do. And then . . . he did this neat maneuver on my neck that he called an "adjustment." It took about two seconds, but all the sudden, I could hold my head up straight and move it all around. The pain was totally gone! Unbelievable!

I saw it for myself. I knew I didn't need a shot. I didn't need a neck brace! I'd had a pinched nerve. And now in just seconds, it wasn't pinched! It was amazing. I thought, "Wow . . who is this guy? This is GREAT!"

But, Dr. King also had to give me some bad news. It was right there on my x-rays. My whole spine was bent and twisted from the bottom all the way to the top, probably mostly from getting hit by the car years earlier, he thought. And worse, my spine had been growing that way for more than half my life. So there I was, only 13 years old, yet I already had a serious, longstanding spinal problem. It was really a mess, and I was pretty discouraged.

I guess Dr. King sensed my disappointment, because he said, "Look, it's bad. And true, you shouldn't have been neglected all these years. But, you have to move forward. We're just going to have to put you back right ..."

So . . . he started.

I want you to know, I really enjoyed Dr. King's spinal adjustments. They felt great. And even though changes came slowly at first, before long, I started noticing that I was getting better. First, my nervousness cleared up. I quit chewing my fingernails and my pencils. And for the first time I could ever remember, I guess I'd say that I felt *peaceful*.

Over the next few months, my heartburn went away, then the tickle in my throat, then the side aches. They all went away. My left leg quit aching. And one day, I noticed: my shrunken leg had returned to its normal size, the very same size as my right leg. I thought, "This is really cool!"

I started sleeping at night and finally I was able to stay awake in class. My mind was more focused, and I could actually pay attention to the teacher and learn.

By the time I was out of high school, I was able to get into college, and in college, I got almost all A's and B's.

In 1972, I graduated from college, Palmer College of Chiropractic in Davenport, Iowa.

I'm a chiropractor, just like the Dr. King who restored my health. I love my work, and for over 40 years, I've been absolutely fascinated with the results that almost every patient gets from chiropractic care.

I've also discovered that some people have peculiar ideas concerning chiropractic. For instance, a man once asked me, "Dr. Gemmer, you were young and your bones were still forming. Was it safe for your spine to be adjusted by a chiropractor when you were only 13 years old? Would it have been safe when you were *five* years old after the car hit you?"

I thought, "Well let me see. I was born in a hospital. A physician pulled me out by my head after grabbing it with a heavy set of stainless steel forceps. He yanked and twisted on my little neck with 50 or 60 pounds of force. Then, as soon as he had me pulled out, he grabbed me by one ankle, dangled my little 10 pound body by one leg and spanked me to make me cry. Now THAT was a good start. I received enough injuries right there to last me a lifetime. But unfortunately, there'd be *more*.

By the time I was two, I had fallen out of my crib and landed on my head. I jumped out of my high chair and landed hard again. Later, I tipped over my trike who knows how many times. I dumped the little red wagon. I crashed the go-kart. I was thrown off a tall horse. Actually, I was thrown off a tall horse *twice*.

Once the fender of my bike got caught in the tread of the front tire, and I was thrown over the handlebars onto my head. In the 7th grade I turned out for junior high football and had the stuffing pounded out of me by the much larger 9th graders. Oh, and don't forget: way back when I weighed in at only 45 pounds, I was hit by a 3500-pound Plymouth!

And now here I am being asked, "Was it safe for my spine to be adjusted by a expert chiropractor, using a gentle, carefully directed force when I was 13 years old"? Are you kidding? My spine should have been checked (and most likely adjusted) after every one of those jolts and accidents.

Millions of children are injured time after time just as I was. Their backbones get knocked out of place so they can't grow straight. Their nerves get partially paralyzed, just like mine did. It happens every day.

The sad fact is: Most of these kids don't know anything is wrong. Their parents don't know anything's wrong either. Or *what* is wrong. So, their little spines never get checked, sometimes not for years, sometimes EVER. It is *so unfortunate*, especially when chiropractors are readily available and are expertly trained to gently put the spines back together and restore normal nerve transmission.

I can tell you first hand, chiropractic works fantastic with children: in fact, many of our most exciting results are with children.

I remember while I was still a senior in the Palmer Chiropractic College clinic, a three-week-old baby named Melanie was referred to me. Melanie's neck was stuck turned to the left, like someone had taken her head and neck off her body, turned it 90 degrees and put it back on facing straight toward her shoulder. It had been that way since she was born. Because she was constantly turned this same way, her head was shaped weird: one side of her forehead was pushed in from when she was laid on her tummy, and the back of her head on the other side was flattened in from when she was laid on her back.

Her parents were sick at what they saw; yet no one had been able to help. All they were told was that if Melanie's problem persisted (and obviously it was going to), sometime after she was two years old surgery could be done to cut and re-attach the muscles of her neck.

Now I was just new in student clinic, but I had a lot better plan for little Melanie than *that*. I was going to check her neck for vertebrae out of place and nerve problems. And I did. And I found *one*. She had just a slight subluxation, a vertebra in her neck that was out just a little bit. I made just two adjustments to that vertebra, so gently she didn't even know. But the subluxation was corrected, her nerves were no longer partially paralyzed, and within days, she started turning her head comfortably in both directions. A couple months later, her moldable little head returned to a normal shape and she was totally OK.

But the scary thing was, if she hadn't received chiropractic care, she almost certainly would have been disfigured for life.

We caught it in time for Melanie. But, what about the tens of thousands of other kids that we DON'T catch?

Sadly, many of the kids, by the time we see them, they already have serious, advanced problems. For instance, a little boy named Josh. When I first saw Josh, he was 22 months old: but even though he should have been walking for at least 9 months, he had never walked. But worse, he'd never crawled or even rolled over. His parents had taken him to the family physician. They had even taken him to the university hospital. But no one had been able to pinpoint the source of his problem. The only obvious thing was that he was getting worse.

When I examined Josh, I quickly noticed that his right arm and right leg worked perfectly, but he couldn't move his left arm or leg at all. The other thing I saw was that the muscles in both his left arm and leg were like soup, almost liquefied with no substance. The only solid things at all in his arm and in his leg were the bones.

I want you to picture how bad he was. When he was on his back and his parents lifted up his left leg and let it go, it fell like a rock (bumpf) onto the exam table and bounced like, if you can picture a skinny balloon that clowns tie into animals and things, picture a skinny balloon like that filled with water and then dropped. That's how his leg was. Same with his arm: he had no control over his left arm or left leg whatsoever. The muscles were just mush and he was in serious trouble.

I began looking for the *cause* of Josh's problem. It turned out that his top vertebra was out of place. In fact, it was so badly out of place that there was pressure *directly on his spinal cord*, and it was so severe that here he was, 22 months old, and his left arm and left leg were worse than paralyzed, *they were deteriorating*.

I carefully began making the right adjustments; I started moving his spine back into alignment.

The results were very dramatic: in less than a week, Josh could move his arm and leg. Within a month, he was rolling over. He pretty much skipped crawling, and went straight to standing at the edge of the couch and moving along the cushions.

Three and a half months after we met, Josh was walking, and in six months, you couldn't tell anything had ever been wrong.

Now I'd like you to think about something. Suppose we hadn't restored Josh's nerve transmission, and suppose he had developed a cancer or kidney disease or lung disease as many kids do. Where would you guess the disease would have struck, on the *right* side of his body where everything worked perfectly, and where the brain messages were getting through and controlling his functions and regeneration perfectly? OR would one of these diseases more likely have struck the *left* side of his body, where his cells were NOT getting the vital messages from the brain, where his tissues were deteriorating? It's not hard to figure out the answer, is it?

The fact is, short-circuited nerves are a serious matter. It's impossible for your child to enjoy his or her full, normal, healthy potential if vertebrae are out of place and nerves are choked off.

By the way, Josh's parents couldn't remember him ever having an accident. So how did he get his vertebra out of place *so severely* that the whole side of his body was paralyzed and deteriorating?

If I were to make an educated guess, I would say the most likely source of all this was a birth injury. After all, this isn't uncommon. Outspoken medical authorities tell us that *many* babies get their necks damaged during delivery. These babies are small and delicate, yet they are being pulled and twisted with the type of force you'd use to wrench a fencepost out of the ground.

The bottom line is, get your children checked *now* by a competent chiropractor, and then checked regularly thereafter. Chiropractors are the only ones trained to locate and correct what I've just described above. So please, don't let this happen to your child.

The Obesity And Diabetes Epidemics

As I AM STARTING to write on this topic, it's early afternoon on a school day and I happen to be in coffee shop. About 20 minutes ago, nine kids about 13 years old came in. During these 20 minutes, I just watched them consume about four pounds of candy, a dozen doughnuts and roughly two gallons of some mysteriously red chemical beverage. Five of them are overweight and most likely headed toward worsening weight issues and eventual diabetes. All of them were making themselves sick.

Currently, kids are consuming 32 teaspoons of sugar per day and more than 56 gallons of soda per year! In the USA and Canada, we are literally watching a diabetes/obesity epidemic unfold right before our eyes.

I'm going to assume you've seen what I've seen and therefore I'll get right into what is causing this.

The short version is that our "food" is loaded with sugars and other carbohydrates. Kids start out early with fake baby formula, solid baby foods loaded with modified starches and beverages that are high in sugar (including natural ones like apple juice). Most Americans are unable to burn fats (the best fuel source) because they've been on sugars and other carbs all their lives. That is the challenge.

Kids are truly at risk from the foods they are eating, greatly increasing the likelihood of them having heart disease, cancer, diabetes, hormone difficulties, depression, joint trouble, allergies and more.

Preventing this situation is easier than reversing it. Simply keep sugar, pasta, bread, doughnuts, cake and sweet beverages to a minimum from the start. It might be entertaining to watch a one or two-year-old eating fistfuls of birthday cake, but the photo isn't worth the damage that's caused. Remember, once a kid has experienced mega-sweets, it is hard to get them to go back to real food.

For those of you who have a baby or child that is not yet a sugar/carb junkie, let me explain what it takes to reverse this so you know why you want to avoid this situation.

First, a person must go cold turkey off all sugars and other carbs. This includes all juices, raisins, bread, spaghetti, potatoes, hamburger buns, crackers, milk and even all fruits. This stage is very tough. It may only last as little as two or three weeks, but many of the tougher sugar junkies need to be off it all for perhaps a couple months.

During this time, this person should instead eat meat, poultry and non-farmed fish plus lots of non-starchy vegetables. One can also eat considerable amounts of organic eggs, avocados, coconut oil and nuts. To make this stage a lot easier, you may want to get ketones that you and your child can drink. (Let me know if you'd like more information on this.)

After somewhere between two and five weeks, a person will one day make the shift from sugar/carb burner to fat burner. From that point on, this person should eat lots of healthy fats including avocados, nuts, coconut oils and eggs as mentioned above. But now healthy fats from animal sources can be included such as butter, cheese and cream.

As a person looks at tackling this challenge, it helps to know that the consumption of sugar and other carbohydrates is one of the most significant causes of obesity and diabetes, and both are about as addicting as cocaine.

If you want to avoid a lifetime of shots and pills and diseases in your child (and yourself), prevent this problem. If I got to you or your child too late, you will need to handle the cause at the root. It isn't easy. But it is totally worth it.

A second major cause of obesity is nutritionally empty food. For many thousands of years, all vegetables, seeds, nuts and fruits consumed by humans grew in mineral rich soil.

Unfortunately, this is not true of commercially farmed crops. As detailed in Chapter 6, most crops today are grown in overworked, mineral-depleted dirt. To make matters worse, the feed consumed by farm animals is also grown in that same depleted dirt, which in turn causes animal products to also lack many things humans used to get from consuming meats and produce.

This situation is a major cause of obesity because people tend to eat until they get the needed nutrients and minerals from their food. If some of these are not adequately present, people will have cravings and continue to eat.

A third cause of obesity is abnormal hormone levels. More on this topic soon.

What Is Causing All The Allergies, Asthma And Autoimmunity?

APPROXIMATELY 16 OF THE most common vaccine ingredients are allergens. As such, they are prime causes of allergies, autoimmunity and asthma. The changes in a baby that result from these allergens frequently last for a lifetime.

As most of us know, all drugs cause adverse reactions including *allergic* reactions. But vaccines are worse than other medicines because vaccinations are administered to babies who are *well*, not to treat something. Their systems are not mature enough to deal with these poisons. These well babies can then have reactions that are serious or even fatal. The vaccine inserts tell doctors to not give the vaccination if the subject baby is allergic to any of the ingredients. Unfortunately, what doctor or parent could possibly know if baby is allergic to these ingredients until *after* baby has had an allergic reaction?

Several clinical studies have confirmed a tie between vaccination and asthma. For instance, a team of New Zealand researchers followed 1,265 children born in 1977. Of the children who were vaccinated, one-fourth of them developed asthma. Of the children who did not receive the DTP vaccines, none developed asthma.

A study in Great Britain produced similar findings, tying asthma to the pertussis single vaccine. Of the children who received the pertussis vaccine, almost 11% later developed asthma. Only 2% of the kids who didn't get the pertussis vaccination got asthma. Another group of children in the study got no vaccinations of any sort, and of them, only 1% later got asthma.

A third study was conducted in the U.S. from data in the "National Health and Nutrition Examination Survey" of infants through age 16. This study incriminated the vaccine industry a little less. In it, children vaccinated with DTP or tetanus were "only" twice as likely to develop asthma compared to unvaccinated children.

These asthma statistics simply look like some interesting numbers until you translate them into how much damage is being inflicted upon real children and the population as a whole. Over six million children in the U.S. have asthma, one out of every ten kids. If "only" half as many kids got asthma by avoiding these vaccinations, there would be three million less kids with asthma. But if the numbers found in the New Zealand and British studies are more factual, that would translate to five million fewer kids in the United States with asthma if vaccinations were avoided!

Remember how I described that NO kids in my entire grade school of about 300 students had asthma? THIS is one of the biggest reasons why we didn't have asthma then and why we do have it now!

Allergies are also easily tied to all the increases in numbers of vaccinations. Since so many kids are now allergic to so many things, it might be a good idea once again to look at what has changed since the days when children didn't have allergies. As stated, back when we got between three and six vaccinations, no one had any allergies or autoimmune diseases. As the number of vaccinations increased over the decades, so did the prevalence of allergies and autoimmune conditions.

An additional cause of allergies and asthma is baby formula. Many of the ingredients in it are known to cause asthma and allergies. Although this formula may sort of look, taste and smell like food, it would be a huge stretch to say it is food. It is a foreign substance, one that babies naturally reject, one that routinely causes allergies. This is especially foreign since most all of the protein in this synthetic baby "milk" is from genetically modified soy.

The intake of foreign toxins passed off as foods continues long after baby has graduated from infant formula. To give you an idea of the degree to which the artificial ingredients have infiltrated our foods, there are over 10,000 chemicals that have been labeled "Generally Recognized As Safe" without every being tested for safety. These GRAS chemicals are *everywhere* in packaged and processed foods yet aren't even listed on the labels with the other preservatives, flavors, colors, sweeteners, etc. Unless you get foods that are real, natural and unprocessed, your child will literally be eating a stew of chemicals morning, noon and night.

Consider this: you can get a quart of strawberry ice cream that is labeled "All Natural" and be led to believe you have a product that may be safe to eat. The truth? There are more than 50 chemicals formulated into it, all designed to deceive our perceptions into believing we are eating strawberry ice cream.

And last, I'm going to mention again that GMO grains and soy are major sources of allergies and asthma. Here's the problem: As with the man-made ingredients in baby formula, we are dealing with substances that didn't grow naturally, things that didn't exist anywhere in the known universe a few years ago. Humans have spent many thousands of years developing the abilities to digest and assimilate real foods. When some "non food" is concocted in the laboratory, a child's system recognizes it as a foreign invader. The attack that follows translates into long-term allergies and autoimmune disease.

Here's one last note on allergies and asthma which begin in infants. Babies are supposed to start consuming solid foods at approximately the same time their teeth start to appear. That would make sense, right? They do not need or want solid foods at three weeks, and in most cases, three months is far too early. Yes, ham-with- pink-gravy baby food may sound delicious. But to avoid a lifetime of allergies, later is smarter.

While this chapter has been primarily devoted to asthma and allergies, its topic may better have been labeled "the sickness and disease caused by persistent, steady, lifelong poisoning." I hope you can successfully employ the information.

Hiding The Cause Of Autism: An Amazing Fraud

WITH THE PASSING of every year, there is a greater and greater chance that you will have a child, grandchild or neighbor with autism. But even if no one in your group has autism, you will soon see that it nevertheless effects you in a big way.

As discussed earlier, autism is a neurological condition where a perfectly normal baby changes from interacting with parents and siblings to one where he or she doesn't communicate, and retreats instead into a state of mental isolation.

Autism victims and their families are never the same.

Autism used to be rare but has now skyrocketed, literally increasing from one in a million kids to currently about 1 in 50 children between the age of 3 and 17 in the U.S.

We just maybe ought to be thinking about what is causing this huge epidemic. Also, before we pass this off as something that doesn't affect us, think of who is paying for the billions worth of care that these people will need, whether through insurance premiums, taxes or out-of-pocket payments. It *does* affect *all* of us. And it is huge!

The big controversy relates to what is causing this staggering epidemic. The officials are trying to say it is genetic, which is about as ridiculous as saying that lung cancer among chain smokers is genetic.

Parents of autistic children know better. They say it is vaccinations. Many thousands of parents noted changes in their kids within hours or days after their child received a measles, mumps and rubella (MMR) vaccination. And sometimes other shots too.

Observers of statistics also say it is vaccinations. For instance, during the 1990s when the MMR vaccination was aggressively marketed in California, there was at the same time a 600% increase in autism. As vaccination increased 4-fold in America during a specific time frame, autism increased 40-fold!

The official stance at the CDC, as well as at local health districts throughout the country and the American Academy of Pediatrics is that there is no relationship between autism and vaccinations.

But try to find autism in a child who hasn't been vaccinated! Good luck!

Consider Chicago based "Homefirst Medical Services," a group which provides medical care for families who choose to have home births and avoid vaccines. They have treated around 35,000 of these children over the years. Homefirst's medical director, the late Dr. Mayer Eisenstein, said in an interview a few years ago "... I don't think we have a single case of autism in children delivered by us among those who never received vaccines."

Let's also consider Amish children. They are mostly unvaccinated. Dr. Frank Noonan is a doctor who treats Amish children in Lancaster County, Pennsylvania. He has said that he has seen no cases of autism in the thousands of Amish children he has treated over 25 years. "You'll find all the other stuff, but we don't find autism," he states.

Dr. Heng Wang is a neurologist and the director of the "Clinic for Special Needs Children" in Ohio, another area where there is a large

Amish population. He has estimated the rate of autism in the Amish community to be 1 in 15,000.

Clearly, autism is extremely common in fully vaccinated children but extremely rare in unvaccinated children.

And yet, the official story has remained the same, that autism is not related to vaccination or vaccine ingredients. But it has never made sense because it's so obviously not true. There had to be a huge lie somewhere in the "research". But until recently, it has been difficult if not impossible to locate the lie.

But finally, the lie has been nailed. We now know exactly what the lie is, how it came about and how it was passed off as truth.

Throughout the 1970s, 80s and 90s, more and more parents saw signs of autism, especially shortly after the MMR vaccination. The first official papers mentioning this relationship showed up in the late 1990s. Then, as the CDC saw that one of their favorite sacred cows was coming under attack, they didn't want to lose credibility or funding, or wonder where billions of dollars would come from to compensate vaccination victims.

So they laid out a plan.

The CDC and pharmaceutical companies had already lobbied Congress to pass a law protecting vaccine makers from being sued or held liable for babies they maimed and/or killed with their poisonous concoctions.

Next, they started the process of manufacturing "studies" that would show no relationship between autism and vaccinations. Listen, I know this sounds like conspiracy talk. But read on just a bit.

The CDC found just the person to head up the bogus studies. There was a psychiatrist named Poul Thorsen working for the CDC. He had no research experience or credentials, and in fact he had even lost his license due to some unscrupulous activity. In spite of this, the CDC chose to employ him in so-called vaccine research. But it was NOT to see if there was or wasn't a relationship. No. Thorsen was specifically hired to "prove" exactly what they wanted him to prove, that there was no relationship between the MMR vaccine and autism. His orders from the CDC were very clear: "Here's the conclusion we want. Make it appear!"

It just so happened that, during the preceding years, the nation of Denmark had been keeping better records regarding autism than the United States. So Thorsen went there to set up shop and to hopefully find a way to cook the books enough to "prove" there was no relationship between vaccinations and autism.

It wasn't long until he had worked out his evil scheme. Once implemented, the total fraud known as the "Denmark Study" was released and eagerly published by the American Academy of Pediatrics.

The "Denmark Study" concluded that there was no relationship between Thimerosal, the 50% mercury solution found in MMR vaccinations, and autism. It went further. Kids with the vaccination, the fraud-based study said, were LESS likely to have autism. (Some of you may have seen the movie "Erin Brockovich" and remember Pacific Gas and Electric saying the cancer-causing hexavalent chromium they dumped into the groundwater was good for people when in fact it almost universally caused cancer and birth defects. Same story here.) So that was the lie.

How did Thorsen and his team come up with this lie and hide it so thoroughly? Well, Thorsen was clearly an evil criminal but not a stupid one. It is hard at first to wrap your head around what I'm about to tell you, so don't be surprised if it takes a couple readings to get it. It is very slick, but here it is:

Thorsen's "study" looked at data between 1970 and 2000.

Mercury was in Danish vaccinations until 1992, but after 1992, it was removed from their vaccines. So, from 1970 through 1995, autism was on a steady rise. (Note: even though mercury was taken out of Danish vaccines in 1992, the damaged kids were already in the pipeline, with many diagnosed through 1995.)

Now here is where the plot gets truly sinister. Until 1995, only autism diagnosed in *hospitals* was counted officially by the Danish registry, and there were "X" number of Autism cases diagnosed.

However, starting in 1995, when the effects of the Thimerosal laced shots were trailing off some (because mercury had been taken out of their vaccinations), the Danish government made a big change and started counting all Outpatient Clinics visits in its Registry's statistics, a 14-fold increase in child doctor visits!

So while the effects of the Thimerosal in the child population were winding down some by the end of 1995, 14 times as many kids started being counted! This (deceptively) showed as a slight increase in total Autism cases counted by the Registry.

Thorsen purposely omitted the fact that the percentage of children with Autism had suddenly and dramatically dropped ten-fold, thus per-petrated this huge crime. And the CDC paid him to do it!

Now, let me bring you up to date. A couple years ago, Thorsen was indicted by a federal grand jury in Atlanta on charges of wire fraud, money laundering and defrauding research institutions of millions of dollars of grant money. He was and is a criminal and a complete fraud.

But . . . by that point, his bogus study had been cited at least 91 times in other papers, thus compounding the lie many fold. Thorsen's "study" is the foundation of the lie still being told every day of the year in every county in the United States.

You might also like to know that of the 7 authors of the Denmark study (Thorsen and six accomplices), three received direct funding (money) from the CDC on "vaccine-safety" related projects. Two of the remaining four worked for a Danish vaccine manufacturer (money). These authors went far beyond simply lacking objectivity. They were financially moti-vated to outright lie.

Regarding the CDC's involvement in this fraud, their own research showed a direct correlation between Thimerosal and autism back in 2004 at a time when a Dr. William Thompson and three others were doing a study. However, the then "Director of Immunization Safety" Chief, Frank Destefano, ordered them to hide these findings and to say that Thimerosal did not cause autism! After ten years of living with this lie, Dr. Thompson finally came forth with the truth in 2014, telling exactly what had transpired. (Please Google his confession and see it for yourself.)

Well, that's the story. It's utterly unbelievable the trouble one of our main government agencies will go through to keep the money flowing, even if it means maiming hundreds of thousands of our babies and children.

I'm going to leave you with four last thoughts regarding autism:

- First, Thimerosal is 50% organic mercury. There is no known safe level of exposure. Organic mercury is the most dangerous form of mercury to human health, especially to babies with developing nervous systems. If a workplace environment was causing a grown man to take in the amount of organic mercury found in just one of these vaccinations, that workplace would be shut down by the EPA. Thimerosal has been out of British vaccinations since 2005 due to its obvious dangers. So why is it still in a dozen of the vaccines that will be given millions of times to American children this year? The older readers will remember the red liquid "Merthiolate" that our parents put on cuts and scrapes fifty years ago, the stuff in the bottle with the "skull and crossbones label" indicating that it was super poisonous? That is Thimerosal!

- Second, I challenge you to please Google:

  iaomt.org/TestFoundation/autismhg.htm

Scroll down about half way in the document and you will find a list of about 80 symptoms of mercury toxicity. Right beside these, there is an almost identical list, the symptoms of autism. Coincidence? Please see it for yourself.

- Third, autism is still on the rise, with some authorities saying one in 25 are now affected or will be soon. On top of the tough life each person with autism and his family will face, there is the cost in dollars. We are quickly headed toward a multi-trillion-dollar problem.

- Fourth, the mercury (thimerosal) is most likely only part of the problem. It is now known that aluminum augments the ill effects of mercury, and many scientists now believe that aluminum alone may be even worse than mercury! Further, the detergent found in many vaccinations breaks down the blood-brain barrier, thus allowing these poisons easier entry into the brain.

Remember that your child's health, safety and life are dependent on you becoming educated. You simply cannot trust what we are told by those who are financially motivated to not tell the truth. The lie that vaccinations don't cause autism is just that, a lie. This lie is damaging and debilitating thousands and thousands of kids. It is an immense crime.

I hope you pass the message on.

Why Are Children's Hormones So Mixed Up?

As I MENTIONED EARLIER, children have fouled up hormones like never before. I was going to call this section "hormone imbalances" but that doesn't really describe what is taking place. Their hormone levels are just *wrong*.

There are two main places where this shows up, and each is easily seen without a microscope or lab test.

The first is that girls are starting their female cycles very early, some by age seven or eight, and in fact, some of them are as physically developed by age 12 as their moms.

The other "hard to miss" sign of fouled hormones is that many boys are less masculine, and many girls are less feminine today. It is even said that hundreds of thousands of kids now have a nagging feeling they are in a body of the wrong gender.

Believe me, these situations did not exist when I was ten or fifteen years old. Whether this strikes you as normal in today's world or not, it would be hard to contend that we are not witnessing a huge hormonal and physiological shift.

Another hormonal phenomenon that is drawing more and more

attention is the rate of infertility in couples, now estimated at one in five.

Let's look at some of the more glaring causes of this hormone chaos.

First, all plastic emits chemicals which mimic sex hormones, and these enter our children via several different avenues. For instance, plastic comes in direct contact with our food and water today with ever increasing frequency. We have fast food containers and water bottles. Water pipes in many new dwellings are plastic. Food is often packaged in plastic at the grocery and is stored in plastic in our refrigerators. All contact between plastic and products we consume is fouling our hormones. This also includes Teflon pans.

Second, commercially grown beef, pork and poultry, as well as animal products such as butter, cheese, eggs and yogurt can all have unnatural hormones that translate into abnormal human hormone levels. Farmed fish too. Dairy cows are given the rBGH (also called rBST) lab-created hormone to make them have huge udders at a younger age, so they put out *gallons* of additional milk per day. The FDA, the American Cancer Society and the dairy industry have the nerve to tell us this doesn't impact human hormone levels, an assertion that is very questionable.

Third, as a result of now decades of hormone replacement therapy treatment and birth control pill use, these hormones are finding their way into our drinking water and *everyone* is drinking them.

Fourth, fabric softener also contains hormone disruptors, chemicals that that can keep your child's hormones off tilt.

Abnormal hormones are related to many unpleasant conditions, even cancer. Yes, it is getting more difficult with every passing year, but make every effort to avoid these factors that alter your child's hormones.

∽ *Thirty-Third Chapter* ∾

The Truth About Childhood Cancer

I MENTIONED EARLIER that I could quickly list half a dozen causes of childhood cancer. Here are that many and more:

Anything that alters hormones levels from normal (and everything I listed in the "Hormone" section immediately preceding this section is included) can not only change physical and functional characteristics, it can also cause cancer, especially reproductive cancer. For instance, the hormone rBGH/rBST given to cows is already listed as a probable cause of cancer, including that of breast and prostate. Please take another look at the "hormone" chapter, but this time with cancer in mind.

Many of the food additives such as artificial colors, flavors, enhancers and preservatives are well known for causing cancer. So are most of the fake sweeteners.

Roundup, the weed killer, is a well-known cancer causer. The most recent numbers I could find for use in the United States was from 2014. At that time, we were already dumping upward of 276,000,000 pounds per year onto our farm soil. That much or more was added the next year and the next and the next. And this is just one of many agricultural products that can cause cancer. In 2018, the courts gave the go ahead on a $285,000,000 lawsuit against Monsanto (now Bayer) for the cancer they have already caused through Roundup and glyphosate.

As Roundup and other farm chemicals build up in the soil year after year, its presence in our foods is virtually guaranteed, and at higher concentrations with every passing crop. Roundup is also sprayed on most grass and grain. We can then be poisoned gradually by eating the grains directly, like in breakfast cereals or bread. Or, when the grass or grains are fed to animals, the cancer-causing agents are concentrated 50 to 100-fold in the meat, giving us industrial scale levels of cancer-causing poison. Also, when sugar beets are grown in fields laced with Roundup and other toxic chemicals, they soak it up, bringing added cancer-causing factors to all the sugar, syrup and boxed breakfast cereals we are gobbling down.

The vaccine ingredient formaldehyde is well known as a cancer-causing agent. This is easy to check for yourself. Simply search "does formaldehyde cause cancer?" followed by "formaldehyde in vaccinations." You'll see that there is supposedly only a small amount in vaccines. But by the time a tiny baby has had multiple vaccine doses containing it, the small amount isn't so small. And formaldehyde is by no means the only cancer-causing ingredient in vaccinations.

And a list of cancer-causing agents wouldn't be complete without all the chemical products around our home. Make sure dish and dishwasher detergent is very thoroughly rinsed off every eating utensil, pan, kettle and food storage container. Be sure the flame-retardant pajamas are washed several times before you let your child sleep in them (and it is wise to always give every laundry load an extra rinse). Don't let your little girl bathe in cancer causing bubble bath water. Avoid baby powder when changing diapers, especially in the little girls. Keep all those "room fresheners" sprays out of your home and the scented "car freshener" products out of your car. Even avoid scented candles.

All sorts of cleaning products are harmful in a number of ways including acting as carcinogens.

Avoid carcinogenic products that go directly onto your child's skin, products such as sun screens and lotions.

You know that lovely bubble gum flavored fluoride that your dentist wants you to give to your child, the fluoride toothpaste and the fluoride in drinking water (including the fluoride "enhanced" baby water sold at the local drug stores)? Yep, ALL fluoride is among the causes of cancer.

Insecticide sprays used on all sorts of fruit, vegetable and grain crops are known carcinogens. In fact, farm workers who are around these sprays have high rates of cancer, as do their kids who are around the toxins they carry home on their clothes and skin.

One of the most dangerous causes of childhood cancer is chemotherapy. It is like throwing gas on a fire to put it out instead of water.

If you decide to get new carpet in your home, I advise that you have the carpet unrolled for at least a couple weeks in a warehouse or garage before you allow its remaining off-gassing toxins into your home. This same concept applies to bed mattresses and poly filled pillows.

Last, 18 of the 50 most prescribed drugs in America cause cancer. Fortunately, most of these are not used on children. But don't forget, kids like to have parents and grandparents!

Well, this list is by no means exhaustive. However, just staying away from toxins as I've just explained should eliminate an easy 95% of cancers, and that's a good start. After all, since childhood cancer seems to be such a "mystery" to the cancer society and medical groups, wouldn't it make sense for us to bypass their pretended ignorance and start keeping things that are absolutely known to cause cancer away from our babies?

The Cause Of Sudden Infant Death Syndrome (Crib Death)

ALTHOUGH IT IS A RELATIVELY uncommon occurrence, SIDS still strikes fear in new parents. More than 2000 infants die each year of SIDS in America, the most common label given to death for babies between 1 month and 1 year of age. We are told that there is no way to predict when or who it will strike. The loss is devastating to families who have experienced the mysterious loss of a baby, and the problem is compounded when they wonder if the death was caused by something they did.

The Sudden Infant Death label is given to a once-healthy baby whose death can't be explained by any type of illness, defect, accident or injury. There is simply no identifiable problem with the baby. Although people often confuse SIDS with infant suffocation because of public campaigns to remove blankets, padding, pillows and crib bumpers in an effort to lower the rate of infant deaths, it should be noted that SIDS is not the same as suffocation and is not caused by suffocation. Suffocation is a separate issue.

What does cause SIDS if it's not suffocation or an undiagnosed underlying health problem? One extremely likely culprit is vaccines.

A disproportionate number of infants die of SIDS in the days and weeks after receiving scheduled vaccines.

Prior to contemporary vaccination programs, crib death was so rare that it was not mentioned in infant mortality statistics. In the 1960s, mandated vaccination schedules were introduced and shortly thereafter, in 1969, medical certifiers presented a new medical term, Sudden Infant Death Syndrome. In 1973, the National Center for Health Statistics added a new cause-of-death category, SIDS, to the code book.

Is SIDS caused by vaccination? One major study determined that babies die at a rate 8 times higher than usual in the 3 days after DPT vaccination. Eight times higher? Would that indicate to you that SIDS is at least partially caused by vaccination?

And consider this: by the age of 12 months, American children have had two to three times the number of vaccines that are recommended in Sweden, Japan, Iceland, and Norway. These countries rank 2nd, 3rd, 4th, and 7th respectively in their lack of infant mortality, while the US comes in a dismal 29th. Our babies are dying at over twice the rate of those in less vaccinated countries.

When Japan saw in the 1970s that cases of death and severe injury of babies were occurring after the DPT shot, they changed the age at which this shot was given. Between 1975 and 1980, they raised the age of DPT vaccination from 3 months to 2 years. They saw an immediate 80-90 percent decrease in injury and death.

In summary, yes, there is a clear relationship between vaccination and Sudden Infant Death.

The Story Behind Attention Deficit Hyperactivity Disorder (ADHD)

AMERICANS WOULD BE HORRIFIED if they picked up today's newspaper and it said that 3 million children across the nation were being given cocaine by their schools and doctors to make them behave better. Unfortunately, this is amazingly close to what is in fact happening.

Millions of children, most of them are boys, are being dosed with mind-altering, highly addictive stimulants that work on the brain much like cocaine does. The drug is methylphenidate hydrochloride; most of us know it by the trade name Ritalin. Its use shot up over 1000% in less than 20 years. We're now hearing reports of elementary schools where 15% and even 20% of the boys are taking Ritalin daily on a prescription basis. That's not hard to believe when recent estimates are saying 4% to 5% of all boys ages 6 to 14 are taking it. And according to the Drug Enforcement Agency, it's not uncommon to find schools where over 10% of the entire student-body is being drugged with it week after week. The morning school bell rings, and students line up zombie-like at the nurse's station to get their pills.

This is a phenomenon seen nowhere else on earth. The United States consumes *six times as much Ritalin as all the other countries of the world combined.*

How can this be? Simply put, the giant pharmaceutical company that makes the drug has pushed to convince schools, physicians, nurses and parents that Ritalin is safe and effective. They've also done the unbelievable: convince people that this medicating is necessary.

The drug is supposed to help kids sit still, listen and fit in with the class. It's supposed to help them perform better as students. But even if it always did consistently accomplish these things, which it often doesn't, what are we teaching the children in the process? These young students who are given the drugs *and all the other students looking on* are getting a very clear message: for better performance, take drugs. To feel better about yourself, take drugs. To fit in with your peers, take drugs.

Today, there are efforts everywhere to keep our children off drugs. But our actions are speaking louder than our words. We can't be telling kids to stay off drugs and expect them to heed our warnings when every morning dozens of them line up to get their doses of Ritalin.

There's a reason the chemical name for Ritalin (Methylphenidate) sounds so much like the chemical name for the street drug speed (Methamphetamine): it's because they are the same drug. The drug producer openly admits Ritalin is a methamphetamine, SPEED, one of the main drugs we're all trying to warn our children to stay away from.

Now I know these are challenging times for schools, teachers and parents. I'm around kids every day in my practice. My sister was an elementary school teacher for over 30 years. I have 10 children of my own. I know there are challenges. But I also know it is ALWAYS better to address the basic, underlying causes of any problem. Drugging children into submission doesn't even come close.

Ritalin is not an innocent little pill like we've been led to believe. Ritalin is a narcotic, a highly addictive stimulant classified by the Food and Drug Administration under Schedule 2 of the Controlled Substances Act. Included in this category are cocaine, opium and morphine. And as with these other drugs, an adult possessing Ritalin without a prescription will be arrested.

Studies cited by the Drug Enforcement Agency have shown that Ritalin and cocaine cause nearly identical reactions in the very same brain cells. Tests have also shown that cocaine addicts cannot tell the difference between the two. So sure enough, ask students at any school: many kids pretend to take their Ritalin at the nurse's office, but instead sell it on the playground for between $5 and $20 a pill.

Then, the other kids 1) swallow two or three pills at a time for a wide-eyed drug-induced rush, 2) grind it up and snort it up their noses like cocaine or 3) cook it and inject it like heroin.

In a recent survey, one out of six college kids admitted to having used Ritalin this way. And did you know among certain age groups Ritalin abuse is now generating more emergency room visits than *all other causes and all other drugs combined?* I have the articles and the reports right here on my desk that detail all of this. So I ask you, "Is Ritalin a safe, harmless, innocent little pill?" Fact is, the abuse potential is enormous.

However, even when used as directed, there is the issue of side effects. In several states, parents have filed lawsuits against school officials and doctors alleging malpractice and fraud; parents had not been advised of all the side effects caused by Ritalin.

Even parents who haven't gone that far still can't believe their eyes. I've talked with many of them, and they've often told me about how they were pushed and pushed to put their children on Ritalin. When they finally consented, and the drugging began, these parents saw their children gradually go from being bright, creative and interested in life (and maybe a bit rowdy) to being little more than zombies. Sure, some of the kids settled down, but at the same time, they lost their enthusiasm and their unique personalities. Their spirits were numbed. They just weren't the same.

Other parents describe how their children seemed to get the desired results, but later ended up with rather serious side effects, like nervousness, insomnia, weight loss, depression, dizziness, nausea, headaches, drowsiness, chest pains and rapid or irregular heartbeat just to name a few.

Looking back, these parents remember how at first, there were just subtle little personality changes and symptoms. But then, when they started seeing appetite loss, mood swings, sleep disorders and nightmares, they became concerned, then alarmed. In desperation, they requested that their doctors take their children back off Ritalin. But as withdrawal symptoms such as severe depression and thoughts of suicide then set in, the parents didn't know which direction to turn. What they did know is that they just wished they could have their children back as they were before the drug experimenting had begun.

I was shocked when I first learned the criteria used to rationalize placing a child on Ritalin. There are no laboratory tests, no brain scans, no x-rays, no measurements, nothing scientific that could demonstrate the existence of a medical disease or the need to be treated with a drug. In fact, get this, the conditions "Attention Deficit Hyperactivity Disorder" and "Attention Deficit Disorder" didn't exist anywhere until they were voted into existence at a mental health care convention about 50 years ago. (Humorous note: they first voted to label kids "Minimal Brain Damaged," but they soon found this "label" wasn't very popular with parents. So . . . they made up some new condition names and voted to use them instead!)

How do we know if a child supposedly has one of these conditions? Well, the American Psychiatric Association puts out a publication called "The Diagnostic and Statistical Manual of Mental Disorders." It contains lists of things to watch for in a child to label him or her with this alleged mental condition. If some of the items on the list are observed, well there you are: your child has it.

Now in a moment, I'll give you one of the lists, the list used to label your child with Attention Deficit Hyperactivity Disorder, or ADHD as it's more commonly called.

Now as you read this list, I want you to remember back to when you were in school. I want you to think of how many of the smartest, most creative kids in your class, probably you included, would have been told that they had the "mental disorder" ADHD and given drugs for it if this bogus diagnostic method had been in use then. OK, here it is, but don't laugh. *This* is the list that has put millions of grade school age kids on Ritalin:

Does the child often

1. Fidget with his hands or feet or squirm in his seat?

2. Have difficulty remaining seated when required to do so?

3. Run about or climb in situations in which it is inappropriate?

4. Have difficulty playing quietly?

Does the child often

5. Blurt out answers before questions have been completed?

6. Have difficulty sustaining his attention?

7. Talk excessively?

8. Shift from one uncompleted activity to another?

9. Not seem to pay attention when spoken to directly?

Does the child often

10. Make mistakes in schoolwork?

11. Have difficulty waiting his turn in games or group activities? . . or

12. Get easily distracted?

There they are. If the answer is "yes" to some of these, that's all the evidence that is needed to drug the child. Can you believe it? Through this, millions of kids have been put onto a drug similar to cocaine, and for WHAT? I believe most of the time it's for simply being kids.

The fact is, there's hardly a boy alive, and very few girls, who couldn't be labeled with a "mental disorder" when using this list as the gauge. And it's especially true of the little boys, who often would rather be catching lizards and pulling pigtails. But that certainly doesn't mean they should be given chemical straightjackets.

And tell me, since when is it a sign of mental disease to fidget, run, talk or make mistakes? These things have gone on in every school in history. Do they indicate a mental condition?

So what if some of the sharper kids try to be first in calling out the answers to questions, as if they were contestants in a game show. That isn't a sign of a mental problem. And neither is daydreaming, which educators of the past always saw as a sign of a bright student who is stuck in a classroom with slow moving teachers.

But if you get a copy of "The Diagnostic and Statistical Manual of Mental Disorders," you'll discover: all sorts of regular childhood activities are labeled as mental disorders.

And sadly, it's often the more enthusiastic or creative kids who are slapped with a "mental disorder" label and drugged with Ritalin and other psych drugs.

If Albert Einstein had been born in the last forty years, he would have perfectly fit the profile of someone having ADHD. His teacher described him as "mentally slow, unsociable and adrift in his foolish dreams." You can rest assured that had he been a student today, there would have been an all-out effort to drug him with Ritalin. And he certainly wouldn't have been alone.

In school, Thomas Edison's thoughts often wandered, and his body was perpetually moving in his seat. Another perfect candidate for Ritalin! His teachers said he was unruly and "too stupid to learn anything": hard to believe now, considering they were talking about the genius whose research later gave the world light bulbs, tape recorders and hundreds of other inventions.

Walt Disney would have been labeled ADHD and drugged. So would have Alexander Graham Bell, Leonardo da Vinci, Mozart, Henry Ford, Benjamin Franklin, Abraham Lincoln, the Wright Brothers, John Lennon and the list goes on. Their accomplishments speak for themselves. Yet, every one of these great minds, and thousands of others like them, would probably have been labeled with a "mental disorder" and put on Ritalin had they gone to grade school in America today. Fortunately for them and for all of us, most were born before the greedy drug companies became so powerful.

I hope you're already getting the idea that drugging the children with Ritalin is a dangerous practice with a very dubious explanation for why it is being done.

But what troubles me even more is that Ritalin CAUSES several of the very same problems that it supposedly treats. In other words, it is supposed to help kids with hyperactivity, fidgeting, paying attention, nervousness and impulsiveness. But unfortunately it also CAUSES hyperactivity, fidgeting, inability to pay attention, nervousness and impulsiveness. This creates quite a dilemma: if a child is put on Ritalin and then these behaviors continue or increase, should the M. D. give him more drug because he still has these problems or should he take the child off the drug because the drug caused or increased these problems? Who knows?

Which kids are being drugged? The children drugged with Ritalin appear to fall into one of four categories:

1. Fast learners make up the first category. These kids hear something once, they've "got it", and now they're ready to either go do something with it or move on to something else. To them, the classes and teachers that grind on and on in slow motion are like the ultimate irritant. No wonder these kids fidget and are disruptive. They are some of the smarter kids, they learn rapidly, and as a penalty, they are being drugged.

2. The second category is made up of children who are given Ritalin because either they or their parents believe it gives them a "competitive scholastic advantage," much the way many athletes use steroids to beef up their bodies for competition. This is especially common in high-pressure, high-priced private schools, where parents eventually hope to squeeze their kids into Princeton, Harvard and Yale, even if it takes addictive, narcotic drugs to do so.

3. Perfectly normal best describes the children in the third category. They're just kids being kids. And by the way, in my opinion, this is the biggest category.

4. The fourth and last category represents the children who actually have some problems: they are facing challenges somewhere in their lives. Something is causing them to be the way they are, and in a minute, we're going to zoom in on them and take a closer look at what may be causing them to have trouble in school and society.

But first, you'll notice, I didn't have a fifth category, a category called "Children Suffering from a Ritalin Deficiency" because there is no such thing.

Sure, maybe some of the kids won't sit still. Maybe some try to answer questions out of turn. Maybe some of them don't pay attention. And maybe it's tempting to drug them into submission.

But think about it: what if we were doing the same thing to dogs? What if someone came up with the bright idea to drug millions of dogs so they wouldn't do what normal dogs do, things like barking or wagging their tails? I believe there would be such an outrage we would come close to having riots in the streets if we did to dogs what we are doing to a whole generation of our children.

By the way, my experience is that most all parents don't really like this chemical garbage. Instead, they really want to make wise decisions and do what is best for their children. But the problem has been, how can parents make sound decisions when they aren't given all the facts, or worse yet, when they are told outright lies?

For instance, parents are usually told that their children have a "chemical imbalance in the brain" which is causing hyperactivity and attention problems, and that Ritalin will "level off" this imbalance. What they *aren't* told is that not one shred of scientific evidence has *ever* demonstrated that such an imbalance exists. Nor are they told that Ritalin does not *correct* chemical imbalances, it *causes* chemical imbalances. It is a type of speed, just like the illegal street drug version, and the chemical imbalances it produces cause dozens of side effects.

Another story parents are told is that their child is only receiving a "low dose" of Ritalin, so it shouldn't be a problem. But would we buy into that story if they were saying, "We want to put your child on heroin, but don't worry, it's just a small dose."

Or look at it another way, what do the police do when they catch someone with just a "little bit" of cocaine? Also, if low dose Ritalin is so OK, then why are young men and women who have been on it refused by the U.S. military?

I believe we need to challenge everyone who is pushing this nonsense about chemical imbalances and tell them to prove it or quit lying!

The truth is: some kids do have trouble sitting quietly, paying attention and learning in a typical classroom setting. It was probably that way in the world's very first school, and it's been that way ever since. But we need to get back to the basics, the simple practical things that can be done by caring teachers, parents, nurses, doctors and school officials to truly make situations better, without using drugs. We need to make our position clear that drugs aren't an option, so we'll just have to find non-drug answers.

There must be a better way.

Where do we start? Well, first, I believe we need to stop putting "mental disorder" labels on perfectly normal children. And again, for the record, I believe most all of these kids are perfectly normal.

Now you might be asking, if they are normal, how could it be that so many children have been diagnosed with a condition they don't have?

Sometimes to get the answers, you have to look a little behind the scenes and see where the money is flowing. I did so, and here's what I found. Now follow this closely:

ADHD and ADD and all the variations of these labels are listed as *mental disorders*. But it goes further. If a child has a mental disorder, according to today's definitions, he or she is "disabled." And guess what? The more students a school district has that have been labeled with ADHD, the more federal money and state money it gets. This started in 1991 as $400 per ADHD labeled student, and has grown from there. I don't have the current figure, but even at $400 per student, that amounts to $1,200,000,000 per year.

When I was a kid, schools raised extra money by having bake sales and auctions. Today they label kids with ADHD.

Remember, the drug companies aren't about to help. They make millions of dollars now from these abuses and will make billions later as these kids move on to bigger drugs and extended addictions. So of course, they want the schools to round up every kid who could possibly be labeled with an "Attention Deficit" diagnosis whether the kid has a problem or not.

But it's not always just the government money schools are after.

A mother living in a mid-sized Oregon town recently described to me the pitch she was given to put her son on Ritalin: "It's no big deal . . . almost a third of the boys are on it. Besides (here's the clincher), they buy computers for our school."

This reminds me of another intimidating and unethical practice. Mom and dad get called into the school to discuss how Johnny is doing. When they get there, they are surprised to meet a tag-team panel consisting of a nurse, the school counselor, maybe a psychologist, some teachers or even other parents. Johnny's parents then discover the purpose of the conference: to tell them why Johnny should be put on Ritalin. Because the parents are taken off guard, and the "experts" are so convincing, most parents cave in and their kids end up getting the drug.

When that method is unsuccessful, another more extreme tactic has been used, and this one should really scare you. There are now numerous cases where the "authorities" decided a child should be put on Ritalin, and when the parents refused, the Child Protective Services took the child away from the parents. They snatched the boy or girl right out of the home and placed the child in a foster home, because it was supposedly "child abuse" for the parents to not drug their child. Wow. I remember seeing in a New York newspaper where a boy had been given Ritalin and soon started having urges to kill himself as well as other students.

The parents immediately wanted him off the drug, but CPS said they would take the boy out of their home and away from the family if they did so.

This brings up another terrible fact that was documented in another newspaper article. The headline is "Doping Kids", and it starts out as follows: "The boy had been prescribed Ritalin and Prozac. After killing his parents, he went to school and opened fire in the cafeteria, killing two and wounding 22 others." The article went on to tell how most all the shootings that have made headlines were done by kids taking Ritalin (and often Prozac).

It's hard for me to believe that millions of adults, including nurses, school administrators, psychologists, teachers and parents, have fallen for the whole concept of drugging elementary school and preschool kids to alter their behavior. But then I remember that we're dealing with multi billion dollar companies that happily spend as much money as it takes to sway public opinion.

I'm certain of this: if we are to have any hope of stopping this tide and saving the generation, we must assume an immovable stance on two points: first, that the vast majority of the children currently being labeled with Attention Deficit "mental conditions" have absolutely nothing wrong mentally. And second, that not one child in America now has or ever has had a Ritalin deficiency. We need to stand up in our communities and loudly denounce this. It's not right and it never will be.

If your child is currently using Ritalin, and you're beginning to think "maybe this wasn't such a good idea," remember this: it was a doctor who put your son or daughter on the drug, so be sure and work closely with a doctor if you decide to take your child back off the drug. However, before you start the process, you may want to change doctors. It's your call, but keep in mind: if your current doctor knew much about the dangers of Ritalin and about safe, natural alternatives, he or she probably would never have put your child on the medication in the first place.

For children who actually do have trouble sitting still and learning, here are some tips:

- Be absolutely certain that your child *and all children learn how to read.* It turns out that this is one factor has been identified as responsible for half the kids diagnosed with learning disabilities, most of whom supposedly have ADHD at a cost of $32 billion per year in federal subsidies and special ed costs. *They simply need to learn to read!*

- Make sure your children don't have stress on their spines or nervous systems. As a Chiropractor, I know first-hand that correcting spinal problems and removing nerve interference through Chiropractic provide part of the answer to these concerns. You'll also want to encourage your children to sit up straight and lighten their backpacks. Stress on the spinal cord and the other spinal nerves can affect your child's ability to concentrate and learn.

- Feed your children better. Think about what the average American kid eats: most of it is full of bad sugars, artificial flavors and colors, preservatives and stimulants. No one can pay attention with that type of diet! And in fact, the Center for Science in the Public Interest in Washington, D.C. notes 17 studies that all agree: children's behavior significantly worsens after consuming artificial colors and foods loaded with sugar. That's a pretty important detail, considering American kids swallow a whopping 157 pounds of sugar per year.

- Reduce the amount of time children spend each day watching television, staring at their phones and playing video games. Beyond a shadow of a doubt, kids do worse in school if they spend too much time in front of these devices. Try limiting their use in the evenings, shut them all off in time for the kids to get a good night's sleep and make it an absolute rule: No TV, phones or video games before school in the morning. By the way, here's some interesting food for thought while we're on the topic of television and electronic toys: Next time someone says your child has a short attention span, ask how it is possible then for this child to play video games for hours on end without so much as a blink of his eyes? Hmmm, maybe the child's attention span is just fine!

- Make sure the child gets enough sleep. None of us are at our best when we're tired.

- Get their eyes checked. The child might not be able to see clearly, or his eyes might legitimately not work properly together. Either way, it can make it really tough to pay attention in class.

- Sit down and visit with each child and see what's going on. You'll be surprised what you learn. There may be something the child doesn't understand. He might be scared of something. Maybe there's trouble in the home. He might be starving hungry by 10 in the morning every day. I don't know what all you might find, but no matter, it doesn't cost anything to just ask.

These are a few of the basics. The main thing is, if your child has a challenge paying attention, certain things are causing the problem, and these things can almost always be found and corrected. Just remember: in almost every instance, there are safe, natural remedies that work better than synthetic, dangerous drugs. And they will work WITH nature instead of AGAINST nature.

I don't want kids to be drugged anymore, and I'm looking forward to the day when there won't be a line at the nurse's office. I'm also tired of reading about the severe Ritalin reactions which occur all too often, like six-year-old Marty from Florida, who cried uncontrollably while on Ritalin. Like five-year-old Tim from Indiana, who began having hallucinations of bugs falling from the ceiling and jumped at his mother screaming, "The bugs are going to get me!" Like seven-year-old Michael from California, who stopped eating, was unable to sleep, and finally was found in a dazed stupor by his mom when she visited his classroom. Or like 10-year-old Melvin from Georgia who attempted suicide after taking the drug, like lots of kids who *did* commit suicide. Or even worse yet, like the kids in schools who shot a bunch of other students before taking their own lives.

By the thousands, children have fallen into what I believe history will record as one of the most devastating, financially motivated experiments ever done on young people. And there's no end in sight yet, either. Right now, today, as I'm writing this, the drug promoters are busy pressing for legislation that would allow Ritalin and other drugs to be given to our children without parental consent through the clinics they want placed in every school across the nation. With close to 16 million prescriptions per year in the US alone, and a total of almost 400 million doses, we are far, far past the "enough is enough" point.

Inventing Depression
And Then Medicating It

THE WALL STREET JOURNAL, which is obviously a financial publication, not a medical journal, recently reported that drug companies are now preparing for huge growth in the business of also drugging children with antidepressants. Eli Lilly recently even brought out Peppermint flavored kids Prozac and hired the very same advertising agency that does the various ad campaigns for one of the largest fast food chains.

I don't see how they could state their intentions much more clearly. Plainly, they're after our kids. It's nothing personal with them; it's just business and billions of dollars.

The pharmaceutical companies are now all rushing into this market, each trying to capture the largest possible share of the sales, or more accurately, the largest possible share of the children. As a result, the massive number of children drugged with Ritalin and the roughly 1,000,000 kids presently on prescription antidepressants are only part of what's being planned, which is to have millions of additional children taking antidepressants and Ritalin.

More than one million American children under five years old take a psychiatric drug. More than 8.3 million American kids under age 17 have.

We need to ask ourselves right now: do we want pharmaceutical companies to profit to the tune of billions of dollars while our children go down the drain? Or are we going to stand up and do something about it?

It's the responsibility of all of us to keep children off mind altering, spirit deadening medications.

Let's get back to common sense and work to create a generation of bright, creative, happy, interested, DRUG FREE children. If we all work together, it can happen.

Here's one last warning before leaving the "psychiatric dangers" section of the book. The mental "health" industry is bringing two new procedures to market, and they will be pimping both of these as "safe as freckles" even though they are off-the-charts dangerous.

And they are planning on using these procedures on millions of children, just as they've already done with Ritalin and Prozac.

Although these two ultra-hazardous procedures may show up under different names in different places, here is what you need to be alert for:

- The first is most commonly called "Deep Brain Stimulation". In it, a hole is drilled in the top of the head. A probe similar to turkey thermometer is pushed deep into the brain and then the subject is zapped from the inside out to damage the brain.

- The second is based on mega doses of magnetism. The subject sits under a device that looks much like an old-fashioned hood hair dryer. The machine is then turned up to "grill" and the brain is quietly cooked.

No matter what these devices are called or how they are promoted or how safe they supposedly are, believe me when I say that they will damage your child permanently and beyond recognition.

The 5G Internet Invasion

BE VERY WARY OF 5G as it spreads around the world.

Cell phone radiation has already been bad enough. Kids have their phones with them 24 hours per day. They stare at the screens during the day and sleep with them under their pillows at night. This is already causing plenty of unseen damage.

But now we are bracing for a 5G invasion.

Here is a brief explanation of the dangers. Soon, 5G will be the standard for ultra high speed internet. It will connect everything that communicates or is controlled. So we're not just talking cell phones and computers. It will control everything in homes. It will also control entire cities, including power grids, warehouses, shipping centers, stop lights, everything. Sounds great, right?

One of the biggest problems is that 5G has a short range. We will be seeing more of the huge cell towers. But because of 5G, within 10 or 15 years, smaller versions of the cell towers will be at 200 times as many locations, *literally a cell tower on every corner.*

Because of the ultra high frequency employed with 5G, the adverse activity slamming our cells is immense. As an example, there are voltage sensors around all of our cells that cause calcium to travel in and out of these cells, and this is a VITAL function. The 5G frequencies increase the stimulation of these voltage sensors by more than 7,000,000 times!

Expect to see "mysterious and unexplained" illness follow 5G wherever it becomes available, much the way we did as vaccinations and GMO foods spread around the globe. Therefore, try to keep 5G away from you, your home and especially your child.

Epilogue

CAN WE HAVE HEALTHY children in spite of Western Medicine, trashy foods and know-it-all relatives?

YES! We *can* have healthy children! But they will *not* be healthy if we keep doing all the things that are making them sick, those things that are causing them to have lifelong diseases.

There are so many examples of what *could* be done to improve the situation. For instance, before giving any vaccination, why not make it practical to test each kid to see if he or she already gained immunity naturally? With today's technologies, this wouldn't be that hard to do.

But better, why not quit believing the priests of the cult of vaccination, look at the facts and discontinue most (or all) of them? But again, don't expect this change to magically appear. Remember that the CDC receives over $2,000,000,000 per year to push vaccinations. Billions more are spent influencing many other "decision points" throughout the vaccination pipeline. Do you think they want all that money to dry up?

And why not quit drugging and poisoning our children in all the other ways. If the ingredients of just one vaccine were poured into 50 gallons of water, that water would be labeled unsafe to drink. Or if just one prescription pill was added instead, same result. We need to quit poisoning our children!

Don't forget that we also need to quit poisoning our children with agricultural and food processing additives. How much poison can a child tolerate without adverse effects? Whatever that amount is, we've already gone way past it.

Also, we need to all quit believing the "authorities" who are making all the money from this. The people in the FDA, CDC, AMA, ACS and all the rest have such serious conflict of interest situations that we really cannot believe a word they say. Same with the pediatric association, the giant drug companies and the farm chemical companies.

Remember, we have been lied to many times before. Examples? Try these:

- Smoking didn't cause cancer and may have been good for you.

- DDT didn't cause mass extinctions.

- Asbestos didn't cause Mesothelioma.

- Thalidomide didn't cause birth defects.

- Vioxx didn't cause heart diseases (it eventually caused 70,000 heart-related deaths).

- Statins didn't cause kidney failure, Alzheimer's and death.

- Butter and eggs were bad but fake grease (margarine or shortening) were good.

- Fluoride was poison everywhere but in the mouth and drinking water.

- Indiscriminate prescribing of antibiotics wouldn't cause deadly super germs.

- Millions of kids needed Ritalin, Prozac and other psych drugs.

- A high-carb, low-fat diet was healthy.

- Important immune tissues such as the tonsils, adenoids and appendix should be removed.

- Hormone replacement therapy reduced cancer (when in fact it increased cancer, heart disease, stroke and more).

- Mercury was one of the most toxic things on earth except in the mouth (dental fillings) and vaccinations.

Looking back, we can see what nonsense we were all told to believe. Anyone supposing we are not being lied to now is simply dreaming.

So who CAN you believe?

Y O U ! ! Just apply common sense to every question. Investigate who will make money if you do what they say. Be skeptical in a healthy way and ask, "Why do they want me to believe this?"

Start observing babies who have had all the medical interventions done to them. Really notice how sickly they are and often, how "dull" they appear. It doesn't take a very keen sense of observation to see that there is a serious difference.

Remember that if the germ theory of disease as taught by medicine was correct, there would be no one alive to believe it. Fortunately for all of us, germs can only thrive in children (or anyone) when they are already sick, with the exception of the immunity-building standard childhood diseases.

Remember that tonsils are an important part of a child's immune system, and if they are clogged up with toxins, it's better to get rid of the toxins than the tonsils.

Remember that humans have been around a long, long time, and we survived fine without vaccinations, psych drugs, unnecessary surgeries, GMO crops, poisoned food and breakfast cereals that are half sugar! We can do just fine again working with nature!

As I complete the manuscript for "How To Have Healthy Children In Spite Of Western Medicine, Trashy Foods and Know-It-All Relatives" and ponder all that is written, I am more certain than ever that there is only one way for your children to have the best possible chance of being healthy. YOU *MUST* become educated, strong, vigilant and outspoken.

Once you know what is right and what's wrong, what is dangerous and what is safe, you can knock the legs right out from under anyone who tries to get in the way of doing what is best for your child. I'd like you to get so solid in your stance that after you are done with them, they will wish they had never gotten out of bed that day.

So please, do take the time to get educated. Pre-think all the issues and decisions you will be confronted with as you endeavor to have a healthy child. Yes, it takes some work to consider all the possibilities and to make these decisions. But I can promise you, it is so worth the trouble.

I hope to hear about your successes, but I will also be happy to help you with your challenges. Please don't hesitate to post a question on Facebook at SmartMomHealthyBaby. I will make every effort to show up with an answer or comment. Also, we'd love to see photos of your successes there, especially those of your healthy, happy children!

I am tempted to say good luck! However, it turns out that luck isn't much of a factor if you've made smart decisions and clear choices in advance.

Wishing you and your child well . . .

Dr. Erwin Gemmer